CALISTHENICS FOR BEGINNERS

CALISTHENICS
FOR BEGINNERS

STEP-BY-STEP WORKOUTS TO BUILD STRENGTH AT ANY FITNESS LEVEL

BY MATT SCHIFFERLE

ILLUSTRATIONS BY CHRISTIAN PAPAZOGLAKIS

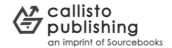
callisto
publishing
an imprint of Sourcebooks

Copyright © 2020 by Callisto Publishing LLC
Cover and internal design © 2020 by Callisto Publishing LLC
Illustrations © Christian Papazoglakis
Author photo courtesy of © Chris Clemens
Interior and Cover Designer: Jennifer Hsu
Art Producer: Tom Hood
Editor: Maxine Marshall
Production Editor: Mia Moran

Published by Callisto Publishing LLC C/O Sourcebooks LLC
P.O. Box 4410, Naperville, Illinois 60567-4410
(630) 961-3900
callistopublishing.com

Printed and bound in China
OGP 2

Dedicated to those who claim it can't be done. Thank you for the endless motivation and inspiration.

CONTENTS

INTRODUCTION: A JOURNEY OF TRANSFORMATION

Welcome, my friend, to the beginning of your calisthenics training. This book will supply you with the tools and techniques you need to launch a successful career in bodyweight training.

Calisthenics has a transformative power that many athletes fail to recognize: the power to harness the very laws of nature to substantially improve your health. Bodyweight training can enhance every aspect of your fitness from mobility and balance to strength and endurance.

While developing your physical abilities is rewarding, I've witnessed far bigger transformations come about through the simple discipline of calisthenics. Calisthenics transforms vacant lots and neglected playgrounds into urban oases of social and cultural discovery. Kids who once had no confidence discover their power through building their personal strength. Burned out athletes reclaim abilities they thought were lost to time. I've seen calisthenics help people who believe they are at the end of their fitness rope finally break through their self-doubt and discover their potential.

So, take note; a truly revolutionary health transformation may be just around the corner.

Maybe you're looking to spice things up in your regular weight routine. Or, you might be hoping to get in shape without making massive sacrifices to your time, energy, or wallet. There are many different paths you can walk along your calisthenics journey, but they are all built upon the foundational exercises you'll find in this book. The lessons you'll learn here are like the scales a musician practices. Though they are foundational, they are not only for beginners—you will never leave these lessons behind. These techniques will help you go wherever you want to go and will never require more than some effort and a bucket full of determination.

Whatever path has led you here, I'm truly excited to present you with not only a body-changing but also a potentially life-changing training regimen. So, without further ado, let's get started.

—Matt Schifferle

HOW TO USE THIS BOOK

This book is both an introduction to calisthenics training as well as an ongoing reference manual. At first, I recommend that you read this book straight through to gain a bird's-eye view of the information contained within these pages. As you read, note the sections that you think may be particularly helpful when you begin your training. Remember, too, that sometimes a piece of information may seem unnecessary when you first come across it. If that's the case, there is no need to dwell on that information, but keep it in the back of your mind. You may discover its value later on as you progress in your training career.

Above all, feel free to use the information in this book as you wish. You can use it as a stand-alone approach to your fitness plans or as a valuable supplement to what you're already doing.

The first section of the book defines calisthenics and lays out foundational strategies—targeting muscle groups, developing good eating habits, and establishing goal-setting techniques—for successful physical training. It will prime your mind to make the best use of the detailed workouts to follow.

The second section is the real meat and potatoes of this book and includes three distinct calisthenics programs. The first program introduces you to a series of exercises that will help your muscles and joints get a feel for calisthenics training. The second program builds off the previous exercises with routines that require more strength, stability, and body control. The final program introduces you to a selection of more advanced calisthenics moves as you continue to improve your capabilities.

The book's closing section explores recovery techniques plus the basic guidelines for building a workout routine to fit your personal goals and lifestyle. These guidelines will give you the structure for establishing productive exercise habits and the freedom to customize your workouts.

As you explore this new discipline, I encourage you to be curious—follow any white rabbits that catch your attention as you explore the vast world of calisthenics. This book is by no means the final word on the practice. The wonderful thing about calisthenics is that it's an infinitely customizable discipline that can be adjusted for anybody with any goal.

While you are getting started, try to suspend judgement about the exercises or your abilities. Experiment, taking time to weed out what doesn't work for you and to home in on the routines that best help you achieve your goals. This process will be a lot more productive than immediately rejecting an idea that could prove beneficial down the road.

Above all, enjoy yourself. As the classic Ben & Jerry's bumper sticker reads, *"If it's not fun, why do it?"*

CHAPTER ONE

GETTING STARTED

This chapter provides the foundation you need to get the most from your calisthenics training. We'll start with an overview of calisthenics, then move on to explore how your training will address each of the major muscle groups in your body. Finally, I'll share some helpful tools, eating tips, and goal-setting techniques.

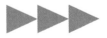

WHAT IS CALISTHENICS?

Calisthenics is classically defined as a form of physical training that uses your own bodyweight for resistance. Instead of using external weights or devices to create resistance, calisthenics uses the leverage you place on your body to improve your fitness. The term, calisthenics, itself comes from the Greek words *kallos*, meaning "beauty," and *sthenos*, which means "strength." So, calisthenics means a beautiful form of strength training.

The technical meaning of calisthenics may help you win a few points at trivia night at the bar, but it won't do much for your fitness potential. That's why I decided to write this chapter: to help you discover a more nuanced, powerful definition. Few things will increase your chances of success more than uncovering the ways calisthenics can contribute to your quality of life.

The discipline of calisthenics can provide you with a lifetime of benefits. Sadly, many people fail to realize this potential because they are working off of a limited and inaccurate perception of calisthenics.

I discovered the world of calisthenics before phones were smart and when the internet was "just a fad." I had recently turned 30 and had spent the previous decade feasting on training methods that were rich in iron. I was also collecting a growing number of aches and pains, not to mention a lot of frustration and burnout. I had reached my breaking point and was shopping around for alternative exercise methods.

I wanted something that was simple, efficient, and would ideally not require spending a lot of time in a gym. Bodyweight training seemed like a perfect solution, but I ignored it for several months because I thought calisthenics was a light form of exercise. It seemed to me like moves you did to warm up or a routine that a coach would assign to a newbie before they were ready for the "real" exercises.

Nevertheless, my injuries and desire to train outdoors led me to explore ways to modify "easy" exercises to make them more challenging. Before too long, my workouts were almost entirely bodyweight-based, and I was making faster progress than ever.

People started to notice my progress but would smirk when I told them I had put down the weights and was simply practicing calisthenics. Not that I could blame them; I used to think the same things myself. So, I started to describe what I was doing as "advanced bodyweight training" or "progressive calisthenics." I wanted to break down preconceived notions about calisthenics that were preventing people from discovering the treasures I had found.

It's funny how time can transform social perceptions. At some point, I went from telling people that calisthenics can become an advanced discipline to needing to convince folks that calisthenics was something they could realistically practice as beginners. Now that the internet is part of our daily lives, the perception of calisthenics has shifted from an easy form of training to an advanced physical discipline. Social media is filled with examples of calisthenics athletes demonstrating seemingly superhuman feats. Now, when I recommend that people practice calisthenics, I'm met with resistance because they believe they could never do things like one-arm push-ups, front levers, or muscle-ups. The script got flipped, and calisthenics went from being too easy to far too difficult. Neither perception will help you accomplish your goals. That's why it's essential to wipe the slate clean. You can define what calisthenics is for you and your life.

Calisthenics may mean the freedom to train any time and place you wish without being tied down to a costly gym membership. It might mean harnessing full control of your body in both its condition and capabilities. For some, calisthenics is about muscle and strength. For others, it's about athleticism and power. Maybe calisthenics is the way you relieve a little stress each day, or it could be how you maintain a spring in your step and some tone in your muscles.

The truth is, calisthenics can be all of these things and more. It's endlessly adjustable and customizable to include anything from push-up contests and 5K runs to doing yoga on the beach or enjoying a casual nature walk.

The Total Package: Strength, Mobility, Endurance, and Flexibility

One of the great things about calisthenics is that it's an all-inclusive style of training. Unlike more targeted training methods, bodyweight training requires a comprehensive set of physical qualities.

Take the simple bodyweight squat for example. You can't perform a sufficient squat with just a strong set of quads. A deep squat requires strength in every muscle in your lower body. In addition, performing squats necessitates and develops mobility and stability in the hips, ankles, and knees. Finally, you'll also discover that serious calisthenic leg training places metabolic demand on your cardiovascular system, making it a great tool for endurance training. So, while the simple squat—like all other classic calisthenics moves—is basic in nature, it provides a wide range of training benefits in strength, mobility, endurance, and flexibility. And all that in just a few sets.

Portability

Few training methods offer the freedom and flexibility of calisthenics. While many disciplines force you to become dependent on equipment and gyms, calisthenics training only requires some open floor space and the pull of gravity.

The benefits of independent training go far beyond simply making your workouts convenient. It doesn't matter how motivated you are or if you're the most skillful athlete on the planet; the simple fact is that fitness success is only possible through maintaining a consistent training plan for long periods of time. Unfortunately, the responsibilities of life often disrupt even the most disciplined training regimens. Removing your dependence on gyms and bulky equipment gives you the power to maintain a consistent workout routine even when life gets in the way.

Efficient Full-Body Workout

Modern approaches to physical fitness tend to fragment the body into many small pieces in an effort to focus on each particular area. Popular fitness routines have separate exercises for every muscle in the body plus exercises for strength, power, flexibility, mobility, endurance, stability, and functional fitness.

All of this fragmentation can easily bloat your workout plan into a costly undertaking that requires a lot of time, energy, and money. It's no wonder so many people cite a lack of resources as the number one reason they can't get in shape.

Calisthenics offers a complete and holistic approach to fitness while requiring only a handful of basic exercises. To use the example I mentioned before (see page 3), the humble squat works every muscle in your lower body while also improving your strength, mobility, stability, and endurance all at the same time. Just like the squat, the basic exercises in this book take all of those fragmented pieces and put them together into a cohesive program, ensuring the elements work together in seamless harmony. These programs will cost you a fraction of the time and energy that other programs require and offer more substantial results.

Mobility

Tight joints are like a personal, biomechanical prison. Just like a pair of handcuffs or leg restraints, tight limbs inhibit you and slowly reduce your range of movement until you're struggling to do everyday activities.

In the past, stretching was the standby advice, but mere stretching has failed to help many people break free of their stiffness. There are a couple of reasons for this. Stretching can be boring and tedious, causing people to skip the cooldown portion of their workouts. Passive stretching also lacks the neural stimulation that allows the muscle to be strong and confident through an extended range of motion. Without that stability, stretching may make you feel loose for the moment, but your muscles spring back to their tight set point shortly afterward.

Calisthenics solves both of these issues by baking mobility right into basic strength-based exercises. The natural mobility fostered through these exercises promotes strong, stable, and mobile joints without requiring tedious stretching.

Adaptability

One of the most pervasive myths about calisthenics is that it has a limited range of adaptability. As I mentioned before, I've encountered some who believe calisthenics workouts are too easy to build muscle and strength, while others believe calisthenics to be too athletic or advanced for their fitness level.

The discipline of calisthenics is one of the most adaptable forms of training available. It's like a fresh box of crayons: It can be used to create almost anything you imagine. It also adjusts to whatever physical, mental, and environmental conditions you bring to the table. I've used calisthenics to train with senior citizens who are recovering from hip and shoulder surgery, with high-performing athletes, and everywhere in between. It's been my personal method for building muscle, improving athletic performance, and encouraging weight loss.

The highly adaptable nature of calisthenics is due to the fact that your own body is your gym. You no longer have to conform your body to an artificial piece of equipment. Instead, you use your body—and its current abilities—to stimulate your improvement. The more you work with your current abilities, the more you'll find your abilities expanding.

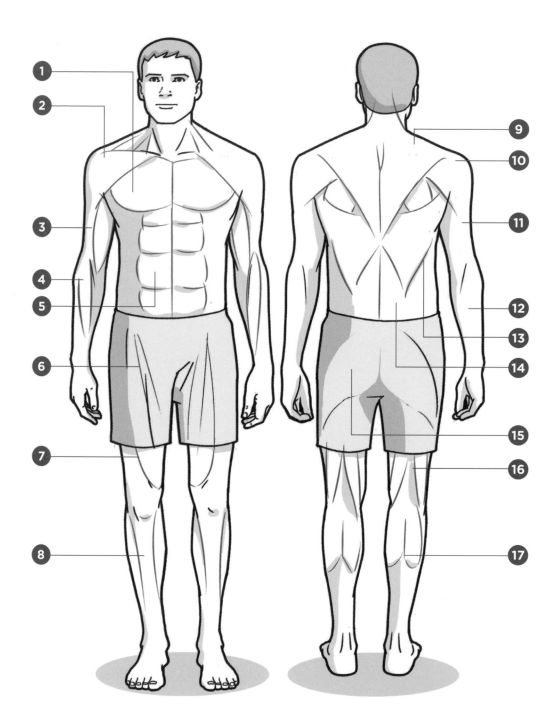

MUSCLE GROUP ANATOMY

The human body is a wonderous machine of natural beauty. The smallest muscle and the tiniest cell work with inspirational precision that far surpasses the latest technology.

Unfortunately, that's not the way most people perceive their bodies. Some people come to the world of fitness with a negative body perception and seek to use exercise to "fix" what is supposedly wrong with them.

This is an understandable attitude when you consider all of the negative media in the world today. But negative attitudes will only hold you back and make progress difficult from day one. Let's start on the correct foot by considering how your body works in a positive light.

We'll begin by taking a look at some of the major muscle groups on the front of your body. These are often referred to as the "beach muscles" as they are the ones that people typically focus on when they are training for the sake of appearance. However, despite their obvious aesthetic appeal, these muscles are not all for show. They play an important role in helping you perform in both athletic and daily movements.

1. **Chest.** Your chest muscles help push your arms forward and bring your hands closer together as when you clap your hands.

2. **Shoulders.** The muscles in the front and sides of your shoulders are used to move your arms in front of you as well as out to your sides.

3. **Biceps.** The primary job of your biceps muscles is to flex or bend your elbows during pulling movements where you bring your hands closer to your torso.

4. **Forearms (top extensors).** The muscles in your forearms help control your hands and fingers. Your extensors in the top of your forearms play a big role in keeping your wrists strong and healthy.

5. **Abdominals and Obliques.** Your abdominals and other associated muscles in your core help bend or flex your torso forward. They also play a significant role in stabilizing your torso and provide twisting motion like when you swing a golf club.

6. **Hip flexors.** As the name suggests, your hip flexors are active when you flex your hips, pulling the tops of your thighs closer to your torso. They are involved in almost any exercise where you pick your feet up off the ground.

7. **Quadriceps.** The quads are some of the strongest muscles in your body and provide the lion's share of strength and power to your lower body.

8. **Lower leg (front).** The muscles in your shins may seem small, but they work hard to stabilize your ankles while also acting as shock absorbers for walking and running.

9. **Trapezius.** Your trapezius muscles cover the area between your shoulder blades and are most often used to pull your shoulders down and back, providing stability to your arms.

10. **Shoulders.** The muscles in the back of your shoulders are used to pull your arms down and back, as in exercises where you pull your hands closer to your torso.

11. **Triceps.** The primary job of your triceps muscles is to extend or straighten your arms when you push your hands away from your torso.

12. **Forearms (flexors).** The muscles in the bottom of your forearms are most often used to close your hands tightly like when you grab and hang onto something.

13. **Lats.** Your lats are some of the biggest muscles in your body, and they work very hard to pull your arms downward and in toward your spine.

14. **Erectors/Lower back.** These muscles run along both sides of your spine and are used to move your spine in all directions. They also work to keep your back stable.

15. **Glutes.** Your glutes are some of the strongest muscles in your body and provide power when you propel your hips forward like when running or climbing a flight of stairs.

16. **Hamstrings.** Your hamstrings have two primary jobs: extending your hips forward, like when walking or standing up from a chair, and bending your knees.

17. **Calves.** Your calves work to both bend your knees as well as extend your ankles like when you stand on your toes. They also provide stability for your ankles.

GATHER YOUR STUFF

One of the best things about calisthenics is that you don't need special tools to get a great workout. You don't need a gym membership, expensive home equipment, or even the latest workout shoes. All you need to do is move your body.

Even so, there are few things you may want to consider using to optimize the comfort, safety, and effectiveness of your workouts. Here are some of my top recommendations.

Clothing

The clothing you wear can make a big difference in the quality of your training. What you wear should be lightweight to help you maintain a comfortable body temperature in your training environment. Dress in layers during colder weather and make sure to wear adequate protection against the elements like sunscreen on sunny days. Above all, make sure what you wear doesn't restrict or impede your movements.

Jacket. A light jacket or hoody may be ideal in cooler weather. It's important to wear materials that can breathe and wick sweat from the body like the types of fabrics you might wear on a run. Heavy materials are not ideal if they hold moisture close to the skin and don't breathe well.

Shirt. I recommend a simple T-shirt or tank top for calisthenics workouts. You want to wear something that will allow full range of motion at the shoulders, so the fabric doesn't pinch or bunch up uncomfortably throughout a set. Generally, lighter materials are better, although you may want to use heavier fabric blends or long-sleeve shirts in cooler weather.

Shorts/pants. Comfortable pants or shorts are essential for calisthenics training, especially during leg exercises. As with your T-shirt, make sure your legwear doesn't bunch up or pinch and that it allows a full range of motion in the hips and knees. Sports shorts, like the ones used for basketball, work well. I've also found that golf shorts provide the perfect balance of style and functional performance.

Footwear. Your choice of footwear is very important. Some surfaces are comfortable to walk on with bare feet, which is fine if that is your preference, but be cautious of sharp objects like glass or stones. If you do wear shoes, make sure they provide a secure grip on the ground without being too big. You will get blisters and risk losing stability if your feet move around in your shoes.

Gloves. You may wish to wear athletic gloves to protect your hands against rough surfaces. Weight lifting or cycling gloves without bulky padding work best.

Gear

Just like apparel, the right gear can make or break any workout. Comfort is priority number one because any unnecessary discomfort will serve as a powerful distraction. Ideally, you should hardly notice your gear during your workouts.

Hydration. This is an important factor in any sort of training, and calisthenics is certainly no exception. Keep a water bottle on hand, so you don't have to interrupt your workouts by running to a nearby water fountain. I also recommend using a hydration backpack since these usually hold a lot more water and can carry other gear like gloves or an extra T-shirt.

Towel or workout mat. Calisthenics training involves spending a lot of time interacting with the ground. Using a towel or workout mat can make your training cleaner and more comfortable, especially if you're training outdoors.

Suspension trainer. Suspension trainers are a pair of handles that hang from an overhead anchor point on nylon straps. Gymnastics rings are a common example, as is the popular TRX. You don't need a suspension trainer to practice calisthenics, but they can add a lot of versatility to your training. A suspension trainer is also like a portable weight machine since it can be used to mimic most weight machine exercises from curls to chest flyes to hip work.

Workout journal. Keeping track of your workout may make the difference between progress and stagnation in your training. The reason is simple: The results you want don't come from following the right workout formula or working as hard as possible. They come from *progressing* that workout over time. Tracking your workouts in a simple notebook is the easiest way to ensure you're making the progress you want.

Safety and Prep

Calisthenics is one of the safest training methods available, but there is still some degree of risk as there is with all physical activity. Taking a few simple precautions will go a long way toward keeping your workouts safe and effective.

Environment. Most of the risk of working out comes from your environment. This can especially be the case if you are training outdoors. Be mindful of the surfaces you come into contact with. These include the ground or floor as well as any hanging supports like pull-up bars. Always make sure surfaces are not slippery and do not have any sharp edges or objects, like stones, that you can injure yourself on.

Grip. When it comes to supports, like pull-up bars, always make sure you have a firm and comfortable grip. Dry off any equipment that may be wet and be sure to wear gloves if the bar is hot from the summer sun. It's also crucially important to ensure that any supports you're using are sturdy and can easily handle your weight. You want to feel confident that you can move your body however you wish while training without worrying about the apparatus collapsing on you.

Straight arm strength. Another safety consideration is ensuring you have enough straight arm strength to maintain tension and stability in your arms and torso at the top and bottom of your basic push and pull exercises. Maintaining tension in your arms, shoulders, chest, and back with straight arms is crucial for avoiding injury in the tissues around your joints.

Observational Tools

Tracking your journey is an essential habit for success. In addition to the previously mentioned workout log, here are a few other tools I recommend.

Scale. The trusty scale is an easy assessment tool, and, these days, many scales provide you with so much more information than just your weight. Smart scales can estimate body fat percentage as well as water and fat mass, offering a more accurate idea of what's going on inside your body.

Tape measure. Most people don't want to change their actual weight so much as they want to change their shape and appearance. If this is the case for you, tape measures are a more reliable way to track your shape than a scale.

Photographs. Photos are another accurate and easy assessment tool for tracking your shape and appearance. Like with any other assessment tool, be sure to build the habit of taking your measurements (your photos) at roughly the same time and place to ensure consistent readings.

Clothing. Lastly, the easiest way to get a feel for a change in your shape is to try on a particular piece of clothing, like a pair of jeans or a long-sleeve T-shirt, to see how it fits over time. This method will give you tactile feedback for how your physique is changing, which may tell you more than a numerical or visual measurement.

EATING RIGHT

Your body is an incredible machine, and, like any machine, it can only function well when you give it the right fuel. Even the most proficient athlete will struggle to make progress on a poor diet. Pay careful attention to what you put into your body in order to get the most out of your training.

General Nutrition

Your diet is a huge part of your success. In some cases, it may even be more important than your actual workouts. The value of a healthy diet simply cannot be overstated.

As with your workouts, nutrition is not one-size-fits-all. Everyone is different. And, what works for you now may not be a good fit in the future. Because of this variability, I find it's better to follow a general set of guidelines rather than strict black-and-white rules when it comes to healthy eating. These guidelines will keep you on the right track while also allowing you the flexibility to adjust your diet to fit your needs.

FOCUS ON WHOLE FOODS

Mother Nature is the ultimate nutritionist. She always seems to know the perfect balance of fat, carbs, and protein. Not only do natural foods pack a nutritional punch, they also offer a great dining experience. Just tune into any cooking show, and you'll find that most of the meals are prepared with wholesome ingredients. Meanwhile, processed and packaged foods are often considered a lesser source of ingredients for high-end dishes.

PREPARE YOUR OWN FOOD

There are only three things you need to consider in a healthy diet:

» What you eat
» How much you eat
» When you eat

Preparing your own food gives you a far greater amount of control over all three of these variables. If you leave your meals in the hands of someone else, you give up some of that control and, thus, sacrifice the ability to eat in the way that's best for you.

WATCH YOUR LIQUID CALORIES

Many people can make substantial improvements in their health and weight without even changing what they eat but, instead, by focusing on what they drink. Beverages like juice, soda, coffee drinks, and even smoothies and protein shakes are some of the most processed and calorie-dense foods you can consume. Swapping out sugary beverages for low- or zero-calorie beverages, like tea or water, can make a big difference in both your weight and overall health.

LISTEN TO YOUR HUNGER AND SATIETY CUES

It's a shame how many dietary dogmas encourage you to ignore or even fight the natural signals your body is sending you every day. Such signals are the truest and most accurate indications to lead you toward a healthy diet.

Granted, it takes practice to accurately read your body's natural signals. For example, it's easy to believe you're hungry when, in fact, you're bored or stressed. It's also easy to ignore your satiety cues if you're eating while distracted like while watching a movie. Nevertheless, you have plenty of opportunities to practice every day, and, over a short period of time, you can develop a keen sense of what your body really needs.

PLANTS AND PROTEIN ARE YOUR FRIENDS

Both plant-based foods and natural protein sources are nutrient dense. This is why I encourage you to include both a source of protein and a plant-based food in each meal. Doing this one simple thing can significantly improve the nutritional quality of each meal and your level of satisfaction.

SET UP YOUR ENVIRONMENT FOR SUCCESS

I recommend following what I call the "stoplight strategy." Label foods using the categories of green, yellow, and red light foods to set up a productive dietary environment.

Green light foods are things that you want to eat a lot of to help you accomplish your goals. Specifics will vary depending on your goals, but your green light foods should always include fresh fruits and vegetables, as well as home-cooked meals that incorporate lean proteins.

Yellow light foods are items you want to eat in moderation and have no difficulty doing so. These are the foods you can have in your environment but in limited supply and preferably out of sight.

Red light foods are the biggest threats to your healthy eating goals and are typically things you have trouble eating in small portions. Do your best to keep these foods out of your home or work environment. You're still welcome to include them in your diet, but keeping them out of your everyday environments means that you have to go out of your way to treat yourself with these sorts of foods.

Customize the stoplight strategy to your needs and preferences. Keep in mind that one person's red light food may be another's yellow or even green light food. For example, nuts, yogurt, and fruit are green light foods for me; I don't feel the urge to overindulge on these foods, and they are compatible with my nutrition goals. So, I make sure to keep them stocked and ready to eat both at home and work.

Meanwhile, snack foods like potato chips and beer are yellow light foods for me. I sometimes stock these foods in small quantities. When I do have these foods around, I keep them out of sight with the chips in the back of the pantry or a few bottles of beer in the back of the fridge.

One of my weaknesses is for creamy desserts like cream puffs. Since these are a red light foods for me (I have a hard time stopping after just one), I never buy them to keep at home. These desserts are an occasional treat like when I'm eating out at my favorite restaurant.

Of course, you may have a different relationship with these example foods. Nuts may be a yellow light food for you, or beer a red light food, depending on how those foods fit into your dietary goals and preferences.

Fat Burning

You may have heard that weight loss is due mostly to diet. While that is not technically correct (diet is just 50 percent of your calorie balance), it is true that most people will make more progress through a change in their diet than through their workouts. Afterall, it's usually a lot more practical to cut 500 excessive calories from your diet than to try to burn them off with an extra 90 minutes of exercise every day. That's why these tips can make a much bigger dent in your weight than any workout program.

Liquid sources. The first tip is to cut back on or, if possible, eliminate calories from liquid sources. It's exceptionally easy to add extra calories, especially in the form of refined sugar, with beverages. Some beverages contain more sugar than multiple candy bars! Thankfully, as liquid calories make it easy to bloat your diet, they also make it easy to slim your diet by cutting them back as much as possible.

Whole foods. The second tip is to focus on whole foods, including plant and protein sources. Whole foods are the opposite of refined foods; they fill you up, give you energy, and make it much harder to consume more calories than your body can handle. That's a heck of a 1-2-3 punch for helping you shed fat fast.

Portion control. A lot of weight control also boils down to portion control. On a fundamental level, your body uses your fat when you don't consume enough to support your current bodyweight. This is why you want to make sure you're not eating too much, even if your diet is squeaky clean.

Of course, how much food is enough or too much depends on your build, metabolism, and activity level. This variation is why I recommend being mindful of your eating habits. Be sure to eat enough to satisfy your hunger but not so much that you become stuffed. Eating at a casual pace can go a long way in ensuring you don't overload your system with more food than you need. This may often mean that you stop eating even if you haven't cleaned your plate. Taking home leftovers will not only save you money, but it will also make it easier to prevent weight gain.

It's important that you eat even when trying to lose weight. Eating too little for days on end can make you feel tired and sluggish, not to mention leave you open to hunger cravings. Such conditions not only reduce your ability to burn calories through activity but also make you vulnerable to periods of overeating.

Muscle Building

In some ways, building muscle is the opposite of trying to lose weight. Aside from the obvious fact that you're trying to add size to your body rather than subtract it, there are some other key differences.

Exercise. While diet may be a bigger influence than exercise for losing weight, exercise is the primary factor for building muscle. Muscle is functional tissue, and it responds to the functional demands you place upon it. Naturally, you can't condition your muscles to be stronger or help you run faster with what you eat. Instead, the stimulus for muscular adaptation comes from your training.

Eating. While losing weight usually involves eating less, trying to build up muscle mass involves an effort to eat more. Sometimes, this is referred to as a "calorie surplus," but that term can be misleading. A surplus, by definition, is an amount of something you have no use for. So, a calorie surplus could mean that you're consuming an amount of calories your body has no use for, even when building muscle. Eating calories that your body does not need will not help you achieve your goal. Rather, when eating to support muscle development, your objective is to make sure that your body has the fuel it needs.

More of the same. The recommendations for eating for muscle development aren't all that different from the recommendations I've made elsewhere in this chapter. You'll still want the bulk of your meals to include whole foods with a healthy helping of protein and plant-based foods. Natural foods supply the body with a plethora of nutrients that not only help you recover from your previous workout but also supply the fuel for your next round.

Protein and calories. The big question that often comes up is how much protein or how many calories you should eat in order to build muscle. Just as with most dietary recommendations, there are many variables to consider that differ from one person to the next. These can include your build, genetics, activity level, gut health, food preferences, and lifestyle. What's more, these variables are in constant flux, so what may work for you at one point in your life may not work well in another.

Some people like to give out recommendations like "eat one gram of protein per pound or kilogram of bodyweight," but these are estimated guesses at best and don't take personal variables into account. In addition, tracking nutritional information can be a tedious, inaccurate undertaking.

This is why I recommend focusing on including a healthy, hearty protein source at each meal rather than getting caught up with how many grams of protein your diet includes. That habit alone will help you maintain a consistent and stable diet—consistency is usually the biggest challenge whether you are trying to gain or lose weight.

Once your diet and protein intake are consistent, you can try increasing the portion size of a meal or two to see if that helps. Just keep in mind that a true calorie surplus adds fat rather than muscle to your frame. If your midsection is growing faster than your biceps, you're probably eating a bit too much and can afford to scale back.

GOAL SETTING

Reaching a fitness goal is like shooting an arrow at a target. You have to be able to clearly identify where your target is and constantly make adjustments to your plan based on how well you are hitting it.

Goal setting will greatly improve your chances of success while also significantly reducing wasted time, effort, and money. The more you understand what you want, the faster and easier it will be for you to get it.

There are a lot of things to consider when goal setting. Let's break the process down into manageable chunks, so you'll know exactly what to focus on.

What physical changes do you want to pursue?

Do you want to lose body fat? Build muscle? How do you want your body to look and feel in the future? Picture what you want to look like as clearly as possible. The clearer you can envision what you want, the greater the chances that it will happen.

What functional changes do you want to experience?

How do you want your body to move and perform? What sort of capabilities would you like to acquire or improve upon through your training? Again, the more specific you can be with these goals, the better. Your body doesn't understand vague terms like "get in shape." Claiming you "just want to be fit" is right on par with having no goal at all.

Do you want to use a particular method or approach?

You can accomplish most fitness goals through a wide variety of training methods. For example, running, riding, hiking, skiing, walking, or swimming will help you burn calories. However, you may desire to reach your goals using a particular method. For example, you may have a goal to build a stronger core, but you also want to do it through calisthenics training. Being clear on how you want to accomplish your goal will help weed out all of the unnecessary options and make your workout plan a lot simpler.

Do you have a specific timeline for accomplishing your objectives?

Goal setting experts recommend giving yourself a deadline for reaching your goal. Sometimes, you may have a deadline imposed by a life event like a wedding or athletic contest. Other times, you might want to accomplish your goal within a given season.

Setting a deadline helps give your plan structure and a sense of urgency. It forces you to evaluate what you're doing, so you know just how much you need to accomplish each day, week, and month. Without a deadline, it's easy to put off your training or pursue it half-heartedly.

Are there any external priorities you want to maintain?

Lastly, don't forget to include other factors into your goal like personal preferences or resource considerations. Maybe you have a tight schedule, so part of your goal is to keep your workouts to under 20 minutes. Maybe you much prefer doing rows to pull-ups. Taking these things into consideration will help you frame your goal within the parameters that will work for you.

►►► BEWARE OF GOAL HIJACKING! ►►►

Goal hijacking is when you start off pursuing one objective but accidentally focus on something else. This causes you to divert your attention from what you truly want as you try to accomplish something else that may or may not be important to you.

With regards to exercise, goal hijacking is an easy trap to fall into because many fitness goals seem similar but are, in fact, quite different. A common example is the difference between a goal around bodyweight versus a goal around body fat. A lot of folks who want to be leaner end up pursuing weight loss rather than fat loss. They use strategies that manipulate their water weight and muscle mass and are disappointed when, after several weeks, their weight is down but their actual body fat levels are the same.

It is crucially important to know exactly what you want and to understand specifically how to get it. Otherwise, you may end up lighter but not leaner, or you may build 10 pounds of muscle but still struggle to do a one-arm push-up.

Always remember that it's okay to say "no" to some fitness objectives. You don't have to be able to touch your toes or have eight percent body fat if those things are not important to you. Be aware that there will be those who tell you that such objectives are important and that you should adopt them as personal goals. They'll claim that reaching these goals will make you happy, but they can only speak from their own perspective.

The bottom line is that if a particular goal isn't important to you, then it's not important.

CHAPTER TWO

THE PROGRAMS

Welcome to the meat of the book—the programs—where you'll learn fundamental calisthenics exercises for building strength, mobility, and functional fitness.

Some of the exercises in this section may be familiar, and others might be variations of something you've come across before. There may also be techniques that are completely new to you. Whatever the case, I encourage you to approach these moves with an open mind and a sense of curiosity. Each of these moves has been specifically selected to help you build a strong foundation of strength, stability, mobility, and coordination.

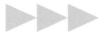

MOVEMENT PATTERNS

There are more calisthenics exercises and variations than there are stars in the sky. It's very easy to get stuck weighing the pros and cons of endless variations, even with familiar movements like push-ups. I recommend keeping things simple by focusing on learning the basic movement patterns rather than specific exercises. The effect of an exercise is due more to the basic movement pattern than it is to the technical minutia that may change from one variation to the next.

That being said, safety should always be your top priority. It's impossible to be your strongest self when you're constantly nursing aches and pains. As you dive into your calisthenics practice, pay special attention to the safety considerations I've provided with each exercise. Never force yourself to do something that causes pain.

All the exercises included in this chapter focus on the following fundamental movement patterns, offering a few variations for key exercises to work each of these main areas:

CORE

These exercises are actually full-body techniques but require a lot of tension in your abdominals, obliques, and the muscles along your spine. These muscles, your core, contribute to almost every form of activity you perform. Health and strength in this area can significantly enhance your overall well-being. At first, it may feel like these techniques focus only on your abs, but, when practicing them, be sure to remain tight throughout your whole body to improve stability.

HIP DRIVEN

Hip driven techniques are some of the most effective exercises for working your glutes and hamstrings while also helping improve your posture and back health. I will caution you: These are some of the most neglected movements not just in calisthenics but fitness in general. They will be challenging and may be unfamiliar. Give them an honest shot for a few weeks. I promise you will be rewarded.

KNEE DRIVEN

These are the fundamental techniques to strengthen your legs and the other muscles in your lower body. The key with these moves is to use all of your leg muscles rather than trying to target or contract one specific muscle group.

PUSH / PULL

These exercises include some of the most popular calisthenics techniques, working the muscles in your arms, shoulders, and torso. The pushing techniques focus on classic variations of the almighty push-up. Meanwhile, rows and pull-up variations comprise your pulling movements. As a bonus, push and pull moves both require strength in your core muscles for stability.

HEART RATE BOOSTING

These techniques may look simple, but they are great for challenging your cardiovascular stamina. They are also an ideal complement to the slower pace of strength training and help loosen up stiff muscles.

Start Strong

All impressive growth comes from a strong foundation. Whether you're admiring the tallest building in the world or the wonder of a majestic redwood tree, all things begin with a stable root system.

The techniques in this section are designed to help you build a stronger foundation for a lifetime of training. These exercises may look basic, but it would be a mistake to dismiss them as being too elementary; they have value to even the most advanced athlete. Think of these moves in the same way a musician thinks of practicing their scales. They will help you learn the basics when you are starting out, but they will also help you become more proficient in using your body for years to come.

I recommend starting here with Level 1, regardless of your current level of fitness. Through these moves, even advanced practitioners discover hidden weaknesses or imbalances that may have been holding them back. I also recommend revisiting these techniques on a regular basis to assess how strong your foundation has become.

If you're starting fresh, these moves should be the staples in your routine for the next four to eight weeks or until you feel comfortably proficient with them.

HOLLOW BODY HOLD

The hollow body hold is a staple for building tension control and stability in the core. It's a **very** effective exercise for warming up your abs and for assessing the strength of your abdominals and other core muscles.

INSTRUCTIONS:

Start by lying on your back on a pad or comfortable surface. Place your hands by your sides and flex your abs to press your lower back into the floor, continuing to breathe evenly as you do this. Next, tuck your knees up toward your chest to lift your legs off the floor. Lift your arms above your head at the same time. From there, apply resistance by straightening your legs.

PERFORMANCE GOAL:

Aim to complete four sets, holding this position for 45 seconds per set.

⚠️ **STAY SAFE**

Lower back stress is one of the most common issues people face with core work. If you feel stress in your lower back, reduce the resistance by bending your knees and strive to contract your abdominals harder. Be sure to end any set when you start to feel your lower back get sore.

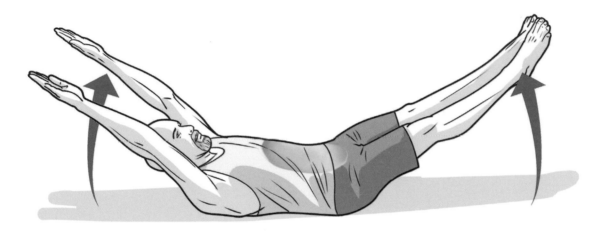

VARIATIONS:

The farther you extend your legs, the more difficult the exercise becomes. Play around with either clasping your hands together or holding a wooden dowel with both hands to change the feel of the exercise. To reduce resistance, lower your arms so they rest on the floor by your sides.

BOX SQUAT

The squat movement will condition every muscle in your lower body, including your quads, calves, hamstrings, and hips. Practicing box squats will iron out any bad habits and ensure your legs stay healthy.

INSTRUCTIONS:

Start by standing upright with your heels right next to the box or bench you will be using. Reach out with your hands in front of you to provide a counter-balance. Begin the movement by sitting back with your hips while bending your knees forward to lower yourself down. Track your knees in the same direction as your toes while you descend. Touch the box gently with your hips and begin standing up while pressing down into your heels.

PERFORMANCE GOAL:

Aim to complete three sets of 30 squats with smooth and controlled reps.

⚠ STAY SAFE	Be sure to keep your heels on the floor at all times and don't let your feet twist or rock against the floor. Your feet should be still, as if they are set in concrete. Also, ensure your knees track in the same direction that your toes are pointing throughout each rep.

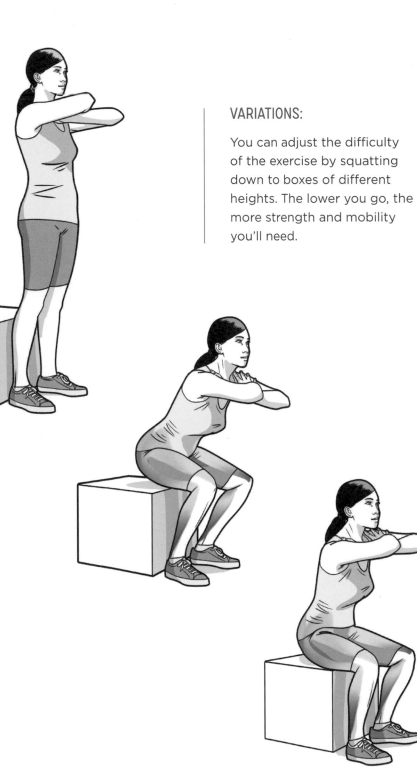

VARIATIONS:

You can adjust the difficulty of the exercise by squatting down to boxes of different heights. The lower you go, the more strength and mobility you'll need.

HIP BRIDGE

The hip bridge is one of the most important exercises you'll practice as it helps strengthen your glutes and hamstrings while also stretching your hip flexors. It's the perfect technique to undo the effects of sitting at a desk.

INSTRUCTIONS:

Lie on your back while resting on a pad or soft surface. Place your hands, palms up, at your sides. Place your feet flat on the floor about shoulder width apart with your toes pointing forward.

Lift your hips up by driving your heels into the floor, making sure you're activating your glutes and hamstrings. Pause at the top before lowering your hips back to the floor under control.

PERFORMANCE GOAL:

Aim to complete three sets of 25 hip bridges, with smooth and controlled reps.

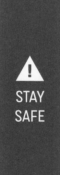

STAY SAFE

Low back stress is one of the most common issues with the hip bridge. While this move does work all of the muscles along your back, you'll should primarily feel this working your glutes and hamstring muscles.

The best way to remedy back pain or stress is to envision that you are pulling your feet toward your hips as you press your heels into the floor. This focus will guide your hips to handle most of the resistance.

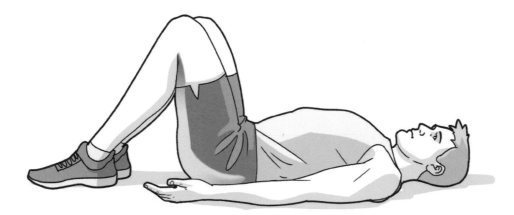

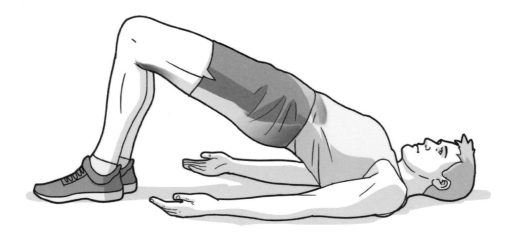

VARIATIONS:

Experiment with placing your feet closer to or farther from your hips. Generally, the farther you reach out with your feet, the more resistance you'll place on your hamstrings.

INCLINE PUSH-UP

When it comes to perfecting your push-up, the floor is not the best place to start. Instead, doing push-ups on an incline support, like a park bench or sturdy railing, offers the ultimate opportunity to build a safe and strong push-up technique.

INSTRUCTIONS:

Begin by placing your hands on your support (the bench or railing) at about shoulder width apart or slightly wider. Step back so your body is in a straight line from head to toe with your arms straight out in front of your chest.

Lower your torso toward your hands while keeping your body straight. Finish with your hands by your lower chest. Pause at the bottom and push yourself up until your arms are straight.

PERFORMANCE GOAL:

Aim to complete two sets of 25 reps.

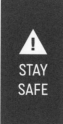

STAY SAFE

Push-ups are often blamed for pain in the shoulders, wrists, and elbows. Such discomfort usually comes from hunching your shoulders as you reach the bottom of each rep. Keeping your shoulders down and away from your ears will help prevent hunching and the associated joint stress.

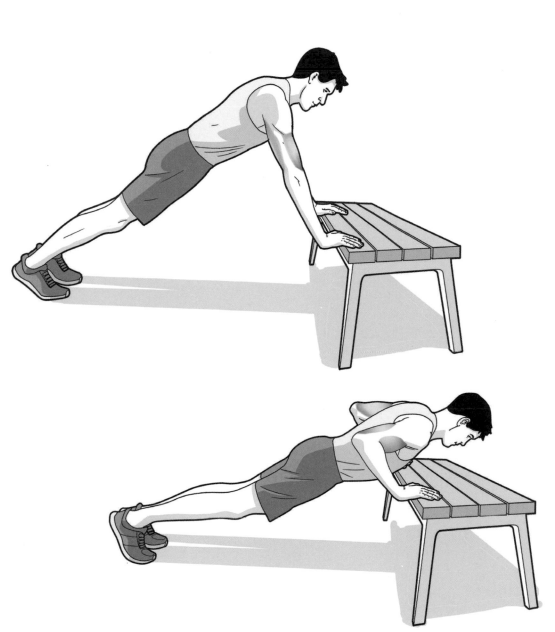

VARIATIONS:

You can adjust the resistance of the incline push-up by changing the angle of your body. The closer your hands are to the floor, the more resistance you'll have on your arms. A higher hand position will decrease your angle to gravity and make the exercise easier.

INCLINE ROW

Rows work your shoulders, biceps, and the gripping muscles in your forearms. In addition, all of the muscles along your posterior chain receive an isometric workout, making rows an excellent way to strengthen your hamstrings and lower back.

INSTRUCTIONS:

Grab a sturdy support or set of suspension handles that come to the height of your hips or midsection. While holding the support, step your feet forward so that you can lean your body back with your arms straightened in front of your chest. Keep your body straight and strong without bending at the hips. Pull your torso toward your hands in a smooth motion. Pause at the top when your hands are level with the bottom of your chest. Return to the starting position by straightening your arms to lower yourself down in a controlled motion.

PERFORMANCE GOAL:

Aim to complete three sets of 15 rows, with smooth and controlled reps.

STAY SAFE

Keep your shoulders "packed" down away from your ears to prevent stress in your elbows and neck.

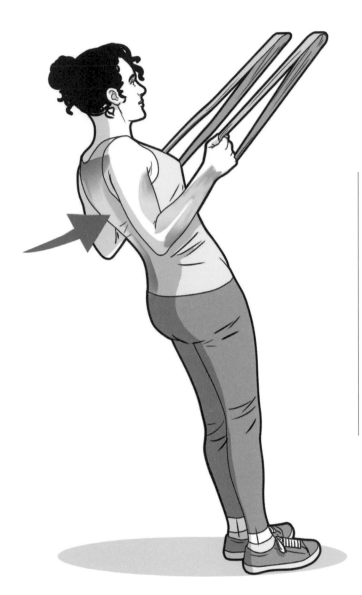

VARIATIONS:

The incline row has a wide range of adjustable resistance, depending on the angle of your body. Stepping forward will increase your angle to gravity, which will increase the resistance on your arms. Stepping your feet back away from the support will decrease that resistance and make the exercise easier.

INCLINE HANDSTAND

Handstands are one of the most challenging and impressive techniques in calisthenics. The handstand is also one of the most intimidating exercises, which is why people sometimes hesitate to include them in their programs. Don't worry, though, as this introductory technique will help you work into handstands at your own pace.

INSTRUCTIONS:

Start by getting down on your hands and knees at the base of a sturdy wall, facing away from the wall. Lift up your hips and stand on your toes to shift your weight onto your hands while locking out your arms. Reach back and place one foot against the wall. Press that foot into the wall and bring the other one up to meet it. Hold while continuing to breathe. Return one foot at a time to the floor to exit the exercise.

PERFORMANCE GOAL:

Aim to complete three sets, holding the position for 30 seconds per set.

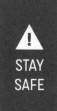

STAY SAFE

Be sure to keep your arms straight and your shoulders up tight by your ears to provide support for your upper body. Also, keep your abs tight so your lower back doesn't sag down. Lifting your hips up slightly may help you maintain a gently arched back.

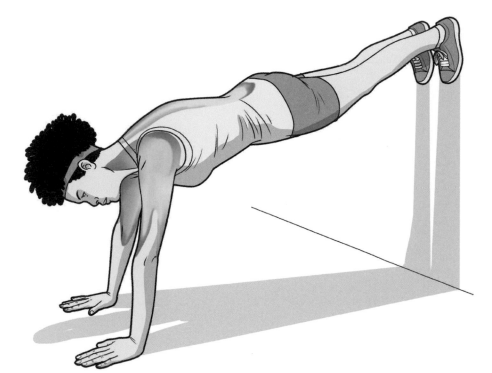

VARIATIONS:

You can adjust the resistance of this exercise by changing the angle of your body. The closer your hands are to the wall, the more vertical you'll be, and the more resistance you'll place on your arms. Moving your hands away from the wall decreases the resistance.

TIGHT HANG

In a tight hang, you suspend you body from an overhead support while maintaining tension in your arms, shoulders, and back. Hanging helps decompress the spine, opens up the shoulders, and improves posture. It's also a great grip exercise and can improve the strength and health of your wrists.

INSTRUCTIONS:

Begin by grabbing an overhead bar and tensing your arms, shoulders, and back. Keep your shoulders down so that your weight is supported by the muscles in your back rather than hanging from your shoulder joints.

Once you've set your grip and muscle tension, bring your feet off the floor and hang while breathing normally. When you're done, gently return your feet to the floor and release your grip.

PERFORMANCE GOAL:

Aim to complete three sets, performing the exercise for five to 10 seconds per set.

> **⚠ STAY SAFE**
>
> Hanging is a very safe exercise, but make sure you maintain tension in your arms, shoulders, and back to prevent stress on your joints.

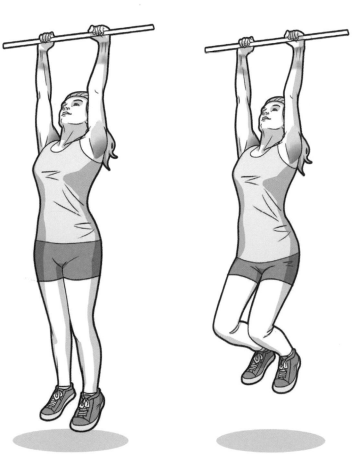

VARIATIONS:

Experiment with different hand widths and positions. You may feel most comfortable using a neutral hand position with your palms facing each other at about shoulder width apart. From there, see how it feels to hang using a wider or narrower grip or in an overhand or underhand position.

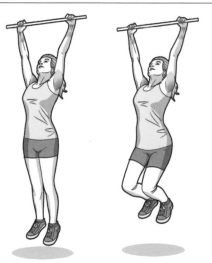

MOUNTAIN CLIMBERS

Mountain climbers offer a cornucopia of benefits. They strengthen your abs and hip flexors, stretch your lower back, and improve total body stability. They are a great way to increase your heart rate, as well.

INSTRUCTIONS:

You can practice these either on the floor or on an elevated surface like a weight bench. Begin with your arms straight and with your hands underneath your shoulders. Straighten your legs with your abs tense so that your body forms a straight line. Make sure your lower back doesn't sag down as this can decrease the tension in your abs and put stress on your lower back.

Drive one knee up toward your chest in a smooth motion before returning it next to the other foot and repeating with the other leg. Vary your speed and pace, depending on what you want to get out of the exercise. A slower pace will help you build more core strength, while a faster speed will boost your heart rate.

PERFORMANCE GOAL:

Aim to perform this exercise for one to three minutes.

STAY SAFE

Start off slow and focus on keeping your steps smooth without any high-impact or jerky movements. Mountain climbers should be practiced in a graceful motion with your feet landing lightly on the floor after each step.

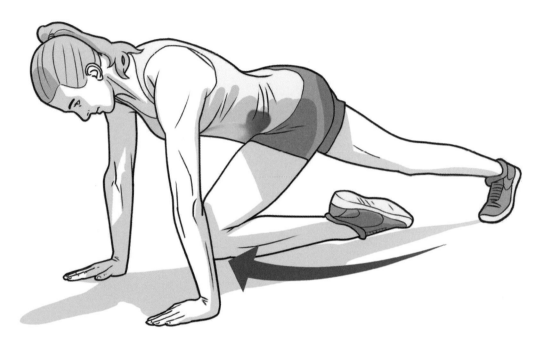

VARIATIONS:

You can make these easier by placing your hands on an elevated surface like a weight bench. Doing so will take some weight off your hands. If you're looking for an advanced challenge, try doing them with your hands closer together to decrease stability.

MARCHING

Marching is like doing standing mountain climbers (see page 40). Marching places significant resistance on your hip flexors while also challenging the progression of stability in your supporting leg.

INSTRUCTIONS:

This is one of the simplest exercises to begin since it's just an exaggerated form of walking. Start by walking with a slightly exaggerated step and gradually drive your knees up higher toward your torso as your hips loosen up.

Make sure you maintain an upright posture while marching forward. It's not uncommon for people to hunch or even bend their torso forward in an attempt to bring their chest and knees closer together. Hunching forward can place excessive strain on your lower back while compromising the range of motion in your hips, making the exercise less effective and placing your lower back at risk. I don't usually count reps with this technique; rather, base the performance goal on time or distance since you'll be moving forward.

PERFORMANCE GOAL:

Aim to perform this exercise for 30 seconds to one minute.

⚠️ STAY SAFE	It can be tempting to bend your upper body forward as you lift your legs up. This places more stress on your lower back with each rep. Do your best to keep your chest up and eyes forward, so there's very little motion in your upper body.

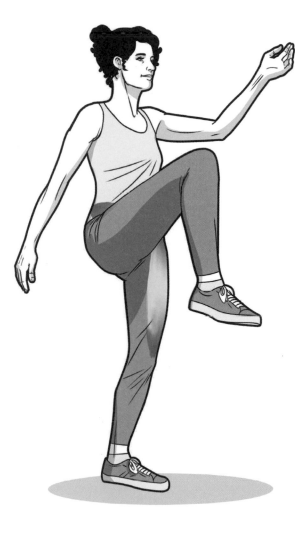

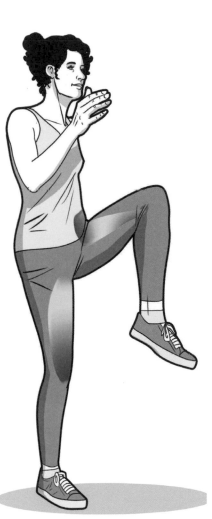

VARIATIONS:

This exercise is all about range of
motion. You can make it easier by
not picking your knees up as high, or
you can make it more challenging by
lifting your knees as high as possible.

CROSS-PUNCHES

Cross-punches are a great core and cardio exercise that doesn't require a lot of jumping around. This makes them an ideal move for those with sore knees or tired legs.

INSTRUCTIONS:

Begin in a wide stance with your feet about one and a half shoulder widths apart. Bend your knees to "sit" into a deep stance and give your lower body some stability. Bring both hands up in front of your chest and clench them into tight fists.

From there, extend your right arm out straight while rotating your torso about 30 degrees to your left. This should aim your punch slightly to your left. Bring your hand back to your chest and return to facing forward. Repeat on the other side by punching with your left arm while turning slightly to your right. Alternate back and forth in a fast, yet smooth motion between punches.

PERFORMANCE GOAL:

Aim to complete 50 to 100 punches with smooth and controlled reps.

⚠ STAY SAFE

Though it is tempting to snap your hands out with a lot of force, do your best to punch and twist in a smooth motion. A fast pace is encouraged, but don't rush through your punches by using a short range of motion. Instead, take it easy, practicing a full twist in your torso while completely extending your arm to maximize the work of each rep. Also, be sure to keep your knees bent to minimize any stress on your knees.

VARIATIONS:

You can make this move easier by removing the twist so you're punching straight to the front. You can challenge your coordination by varying the height of your punches with some low punches—done at your belt level—mixed in with middle punches at chest height and high punches at an upward angle.

START STRONG WORKOUT

Creating a workout is like cooking in the kitchen. Each of the exercises is a basic ingredient, and you mix them together into a recipe with its own unique flavor. Give this workout a try and see how it appeals to your tastes. Feel free to make adjustments based on your preferences and level of fitness.

Cardio/Warm-up

TWO ROUNDS OF:

MARCHING 1 minute (page 42)

MOUNTAIN CLIMBERS 30 seconds (page 40)

CROSS-PUNCHES 30 seconds (page 44)

Main strength workout

THREE ROUNDS OF:

INCLINE PUSH-UPS 12 reps (page 32)

INCLINE ROWS 12 reps (page 34)

BOX SQUATS 20 reps (page 28)

INCLINE HANDSTAND 15 seconds (page 36)

TIGHT HANG 30 seconds (page 38)

HOLLOW BODY HOLD 20 seconds (page 26)

Go Deeper

The techniques in this section build upon the movements in the first level to progress your physical strength, stability, and mobility. Don't be discouraged if you are very challenged by some of these exercises. Calisthenics has a way of exposing weaknesses that may have been hiding in plain sight for many years. Thankfully, these movements will not only expose such issues but also help you eliminate them for good.

It's also a smart idea to mix up the techniques you find in this section with the exercises from Level 1. It's natural to be stronger in some movements than others; you might be on Level 2 for legs, but Level 1 for handstands. Always do what you feel is best for your body and your current level of fitness. Forcing yourself to practice techniques that are too easy or too difficult can pull you out of alignment and compromise both the effectiveness of your training as well as your safety.

Lastly, feel free to make modifications to adjust these techniques to your body and capabilities. Listen to your joints and avoid doing things that cause pain. A little discomfort is a natural part of intense physical training, but actual pain is Mother Nature's way of letting you know that something is wrong and needs to be addressed.

LYING LEG RAISE

The lying leg raise builds off the foundation of the hollow body hold (see page 26). The key with this move is to continue to press your lower back into the floor and use your hip joint for the movement. Not only will this ensure that you're maintaining tension in your abs, but it will also improve your hip strength and mobility.

INSTRUCTIONS:

Start by lying on the floor with your hands by your sides, feet on the floor, and knees bent. Tense your abs and press your lower back into the floor while pulling your toes back to engage the muscles in the front of your legs. From there, lift both feet off the floor at the same time while exhaling. Continue to pull your legs up toward your torso until your tailbone pulls slightly off the floor. Pause at the top and lower your feet back to the floor in a controlled motion. Let your feet gently "kiss" the floor and repeat.

PERFORMANCE GOAL:

Aim to complete three sets of 25 with smooth and controlled reps.

STAY SAFE

Moving with control while keeping your lower back on the floor will help prevent lower back stress and improve the tension in your abs.

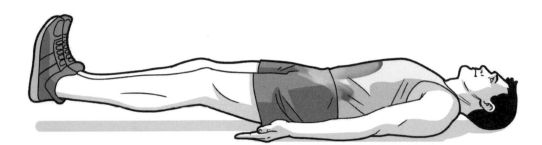

VARIATIONS:

Straightening your legs will add resistance while also increasing the range of motion in your hips. Bending your knees reduces both range of motion and resistance.

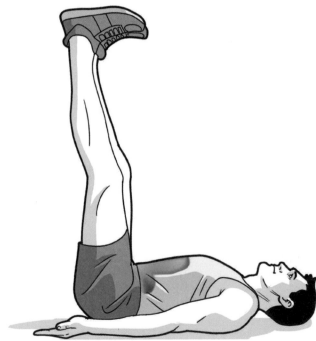

SPLIT SQUAT

The split squat is a great introduction to single-leg training. Placing weight on a single leg requires more strength and stability in your lower body while providing a mobility workout for both the front and back of your hips.

INSTRUCTIONS:

Place your feet in the stance you would take if you took a big step forward. Be sure your stance isn't too narrow, which can make you feel like you're trying to balance on a tightrope. Keeping your feet about shoulder width apart will create more stability. Your weight should be equally distributed between both feet in the top position.

Begin the exercise by bending both knees at the same time while slightly shifting your weight forward onto your front leg. Allow your back heel to lift off the floor and your front knee to track over your toes. Keep your front heel on the floor as you lower your back knee to about an inch off the floor. Pause at the bottom before pushing your front heel through the floor to bring yourself back to the starting position.

PERFORMANCE GOAL:

Aim to complete two sets of 30 reps on each leg.

STAY SAFE

Focus on keeping your pelvis square to the floor and squared to a forward-facing wall. This will ensure you don't tilt your pelvis forward or to the side, both of which can cause stress on your knees.

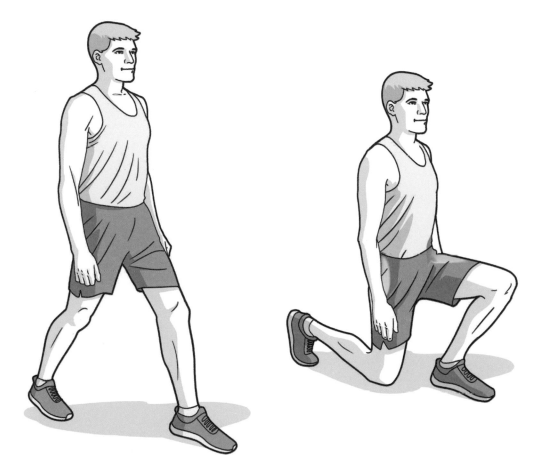

VARIATIONS:

You can make split squats easier by holding on to something to support yourself or shorten your range of motion by not lowering your knee as close to the floor.

If you want a bit more challenge, try placing your hands behind your head with your elbows pointing out to the sides. This position will make you more top-heavy, requiring your legs to work harder to control your movement.

TABLE BRIDGE

The table bridge progresses the strength and mobility demands of the lying hip bridge (see page 30) by bringing your torso off the floor. Not only does this require strength in your glutes and hamstrings, but it is also a very good shoulder mobility exercise that strengthens your upper back.

INSTRUCTIONS:

Start by sitting on the floor with your knees bent at a 90-degree angle and with your feet flat on the floor. Place your hands behind your hips and lean your torso back. Your body should resemble a "M" when viewed from the side.

Pull your shoulder blades back and down, lifting your chest up to extend your spine. From there, pull your heels into the floor while using your glutes and hamstrings to lift your hips straight up until you form a table position. Pause at the top while continuing to breathe smoothly. Return your hips to the floor, maintaining tension in your glutes and hamstrings.

PERFORMANCE GOAL:

Aim to complete three sets of 15 reps with a full range of motion.

STAY SAFE

Do your best to lift your hips in a smooth and controlled motion rather than thrusting your hips up. Moving with a fast motion can strain your lower back and shoulders.

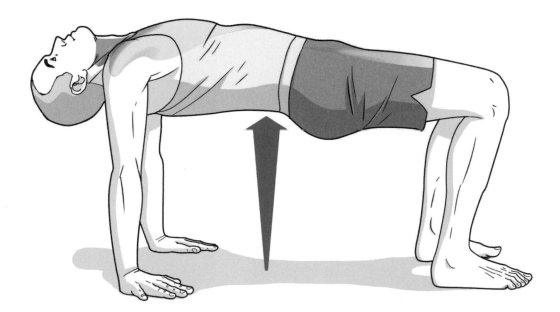

VARIATIONS:

You can adjust this exercise by changing the placement of your feet. Straightening your legs will add resistance, while bending your knees further will reduce resistance.

FLOOR PUSH-UP

The classic floor push-up is the natural progression from pushing off an elevated surface as we did in Level 1 [see page 32]. This classic move is a great upper body and core exercise that will serve you well for the length of your training career.

INSTRUCTIONS:

Begin in the kneeling position with your hands about shoulder width apart and positioned under your chest. Push your shoulder blades apart and tense your arms, chest, and core muscles to brace against the floor. Lift your knees off the floor to add resistance onto your arms.

Bend your elbows back to lower your chest down to the floor. Pause about an inch above the floor and press your palms flat into the floor to return to the starting position.

PERFORMANCE GOAL:

Aim to complete three sets of 25 reps with a full range of motion.

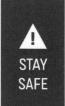

STAY SAFE

Do your best to keep your arms tucked in by your sides while preventing your hips from sagging as you fatigue. Doing so will reduce the stress in your lower back and on the joints of your upper body.

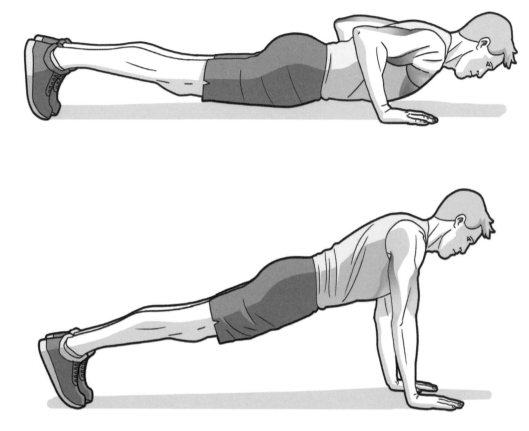

VARIATIONS:

Experiment with different hand widths to make the classic push-up more challenging. Using a narrow hand placement creates more work for your arms since your triceps will be handling more of the resistance. A wider hand position directs more of the work to your chest muscles.

AUSTRALIAN PULL-UP

The Australian pull-up (named such because you're down under the bar) is the perfect match to your floor push-up (see page 54). It's such an effective exercise for the back and biceps that some people use this as their standard pulling exercise over traditional pull-ups.

INSTRUCTIONS:

Start by sitting on the floor beneath a sturdy support that's roughly hip height. Reach up and grab the bar with your hands about shoulder width apart. Tense your back muscles to pack your shoulders down away from your ears. Press your heels into the floor and lift your hips so that your body forms a straight line.

From there, pull the bottom of your chest up toward your hands as you drive your elbows behind you. Pause at the top, then straighten your arms to lower your torso toward the floor while maintaining a straight posture.

PERFORMANCE GOAL:

Aim to complete three sets of eight to 10 pull-ups, with smooth and controlled reps.

STAY SAFE

Resist the temptation to bend your body or thrust your hips up to make the exercise easier. Put as much tension as you can in your glutes and hamstrings to prevent stress in your lower back.

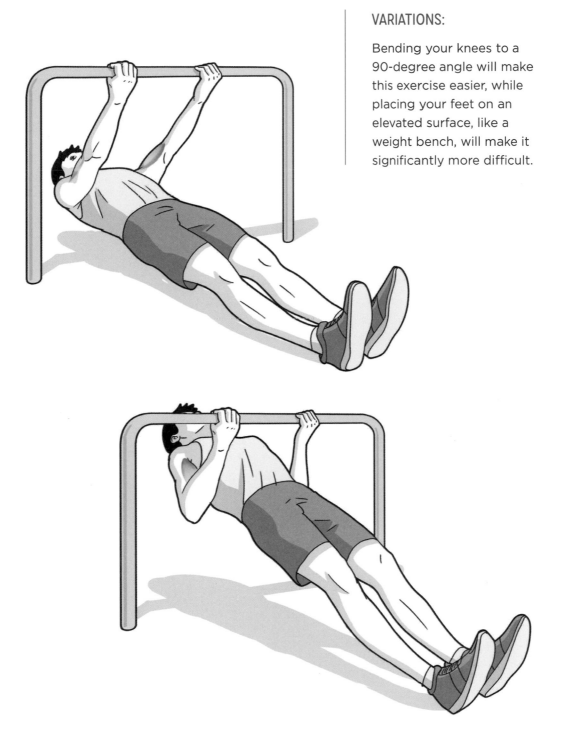

VARIATIONS:

Bending your knees to a 90-degree angle will make this exercise easier, while placing your feet on an elevated surface, like a weight bench, will make it significantly more difficult.

HANGING TUCK

The hanging tuck is a very effective exercise for developing the core control and back strength that you'll need for more advanced calisthenics. It's also a fun way to warm up your shoulders.

INSTRUCTIONS:

Grab a bar or support that's about chest height, using the same hand position you would use for a tight hang (see page 38). Tense all of the muscles in your core and back. From there, push your feet off the floor and, keeping your legs bent, kick both legs up until your knees are between your arms. Hold that position while breathing smoothly. Return your feet back to the floor in a smooth and controlled motion.

PERFORMANCE GOAL:

Aim to complete three sets, holding a tuck position for 15 to 20 seconds per set.

STAY SAFE — Make sure you have a secure grip before pushing off the floor to avoid falling. Lower your legs in a controlled motion to prevent crashing your feet onto the ground.

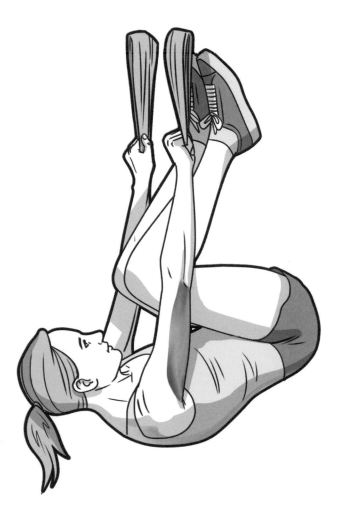

VARIATIONS:

Hanging tucks are adjusted by the angle of your hips to gravity. The higher you lift your hips, the less resistance you'll have on your arms and back. Lowering your hips will increase the resistance of the exercise.

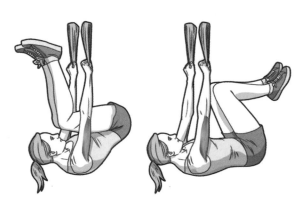

WALL-WALKING HANDSTAND

Wall-walking handstands are a great way to build strength and stability in your shoulders while becoming more comfortable with progressively loading your arms for advanced handstand training.

INSTRUCTIONS:

Begin in the same starting position as the incline handstand (see page 36) , with your hands on the floor and placing one foot at a time against the wall behind you. Shift your weight onto one arm and step the opposite foot a few inches higher up the wall. Repeat on the other side as you walk your hands back toward the wall. Your goal here is to walk your feet higher up the wall as you simultaneously walk your hands closer in toward the base of the wall. Pause at the top before crawling your hands forward while walking your feet back down the wall to the floor.

PERFORMANCE GOAL:

Aim to complete three total trips up and down the wall.

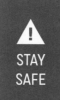
STAY SAFE — Always maintain full control and move smoothly. Never hold the top position until your arms are about to give out; you want to ensure you have enough energy in your arms to walk yourself back down safely.

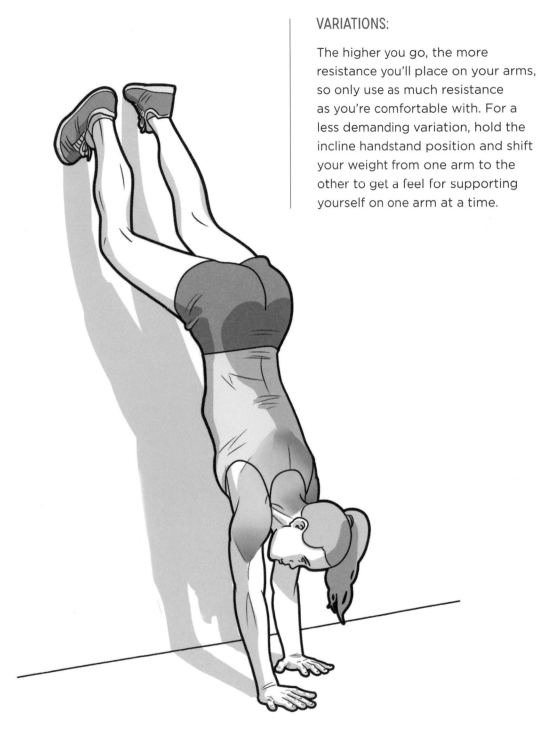

VARIATIONS:

The higher you go, the more resistance you'll place on your arms, so only use as much resistance as you're comfortable with. For a less demanding variation, hold the incline handstand position and shift your weight from one arm to the other to get a feel for supporting yourself on one arm at a time.

STANDING CALF RAISES

Calf raises are a staple for building lower body stability and ankle strength. They strengthen the lower leg to provide extra power for jumping and sprinting. Calf raises are often considered an ankle driven exercise since the primary movement is in the ankle joint. Here, we identify them as a knee driven exercise because, while the movement of the exercise does happen at the ankle, the rest of the muscles in the leg are used isometrically to maintain strong form. Keep your quads, hamstrings, and glutes tense to prevent knee or hip movement, which can compromise the workload on the calves.

INSTRUCTIONS:

Stand with your feet about shoulder width apart. Stand either on a block, or with your feet flat on the floor. Place your hands on a wall or other support for stability assistance. Tense all of the muscles in your lower body, including your hamstrings, glutes, and quads. Shift your weight onto the balls of your feet and gently lift your heels up off the floor. Lift as high as you can with control and lower your heels back to the floor while maintaining weight on the balls of your feet.

PERFORMANCE GOAL:

Aim to perform two sets of 30 reps without losing your balance.

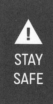

! STAY SAFE Be gentle when your heels touch the floor at the bottom of each rep to prevent striking the ground and sending impact stress up your spine. To prevent stress on your ankles, make sure your feet do not turn outward at the top of each rep.

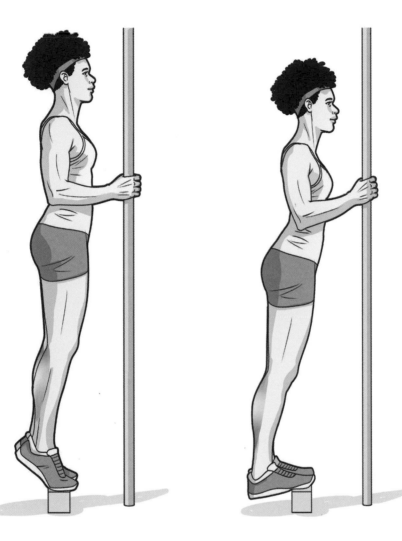

VARIATIONS:

Leaning into the wall will remove some of the resistance on your feet and make the exercise easier. To add resistance, lower your hands down by your sides or clasp them in front of your hips.

SIDE PLANK

Side planks introduce you to a new level of total body stability and core control. They place your body in a sideways position to gravity, which helps strengthen your obliques and spinal muscles.

INSTRUCTIONS:

Lie on your side with your upper body supported on your forearm. Stack your feet and activate your legs. Press into your arm and the sides of your feet to lift your hips off the floor. Hold before gently lowering your hips to the floor. Repeat on the other side.

PERFORMANCE GOAL:

Aim to hold the position for 30 seconds, twice on each side.

> **! STAY SAFE**
>
> Proper body alignment is important for preventing stress along your spine. Make sure your hips are not flexed, causing your body to bend in half. Keep your spine straight and avoid twisting your torso.

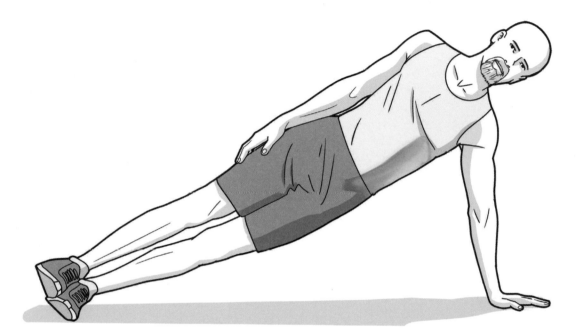

VARIATIONS:

Play with your foot placement to adjust the amount of stability you have during the exercise. A wider stance will feel more stable, while keeping your feet stacked will be more challenging.

ISOMETRIC SQUAT

Static leg workouts like the isometric squat are valuable tools for building lower body strength, stamina, and mobility. The isometric squat is also an incredible conditioning exercise for skiing and trail running.

INSTRUCTIONS:

Squat down as you normally would for a box squat (see page 28), holding the bottom position with your thighs parallel to the floor. Pay attention to your posture; try to keep your torso as upright as possible while looking forward. It helps to first start practicing this move with your arms out in front to act as a counterbalance. Stand back up out of the squat position when the set is over.

PERFORMANCE GOAL:

Aim to complete three sets, holding the position for 45 seconds per set.

> ⚠️ **STAY SAFE**
>
> I recommend practicing isometric squats just above a box or bench that you can sit down on or near something you can grab on to when your set is finished. Pulling yourself up with your arms is safer than struggling to stand up when your legs are really tired.

VARIATIONS:

Try bringing your hands closer to your chest to increase the resistance and instability. You can also make this move easier by not squatting down all the way to parallel.

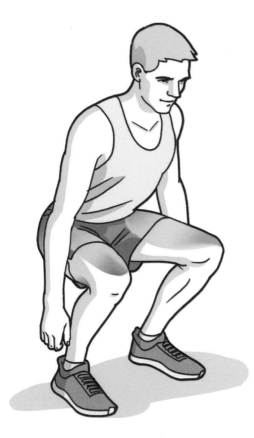

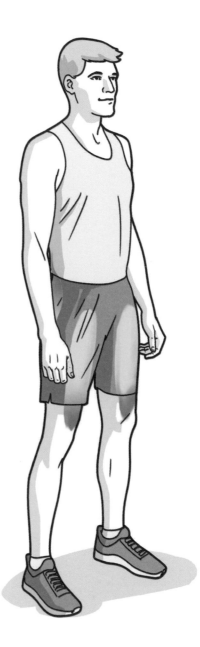

SQUAT THRUSTS

Squat thrusts are a full-body exercise that works a lot of muscles while also helping stretch out your back. These are considered a heart rate boosting activity because they require that you use almost every muscle in your body, thus creating a strong demand on your cardio-vascular system.

INSTRUCTIONS:

Squat thrusts are similar to isometric squats (see page 66), either with a box under your hips or free form, only you perform them at a fast tempo while reaching your hands overhead when you stand up on each rep. Pull your hands toward your torso as you squat back down, and repeat.

Start off with short sets of 10 to 12 reps to get a feel for the technique and pace of this move. Unlike the strength-based exercises in this book, you want to perform this in a fast and continuous motion without pausing at the top and bottom of each rep. Maintain control by working with a smooth motion; avoid jerky stops so that you don't overstress your joints.

PERFORMANCE GOAL:

Aim to complete 10 to 20 reps with smooth and controlled reps.

STAY SAFE
The biggest risk of this move comes from bending forward as you squat down. It's important to keep your torso as upright as possible to prevent stress in your lower back.

VARIATIONS:

Like many squatting movements, this technique is more challenging the deeper you squat, so adjust the depth of your squat as necessary for your fitness level. You can also squat down to a bench or step to give yourself a definitive stopping point at the bottom of each rep.

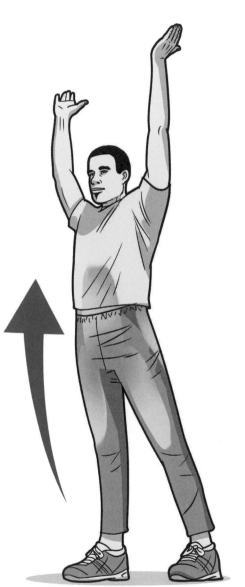

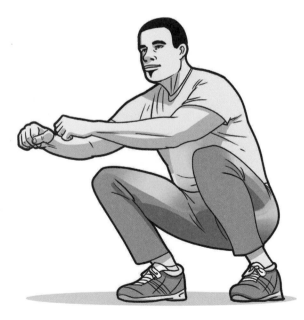

STEP-UPS

When it comes to cardio, nothing beats climbing a big hill or a flight of stairs. However, you may not have access to a long and steep incline, so you can simulate the process with stationary step-ups.

INSTRUCTIONS:

You can practice step-ups two ways. The first is to start on the floor in front of a step. Step up onto it one foot at a time. From there, step back down onto the floor one foot at a time and repeat. You may want to alternate which foot steps up first, or you can stick to stepping up with one leg, and then do the opposite in the next set.

The second technique is to start on top of the step and step down with just one foot while keeping the other one on the step. Return the foot on the floor back to the step and repeat on the other side. This technique ensures you're always stepping up or down and not getting a second to rest back on the floor.

PERFORMANCE GOAL:

Aim to perform this exercise for one to two minutes for each set.

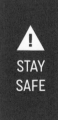

STAY SAFE

I highly recommend using a step that's not too high, so you don't feel like you're falling backward when you step down. You'll always want to step down in a controlled manner to avoid risking a misstep or a turned ankle. A step that's eight to 12 inches high should be fine for most people.

VARIATIONS:

Try performing this exercise while keeping your knees bent, so you maintain constant tension in your legs. Straightening your legs at the top and bottom of each step gives your muscles a momentary rest.

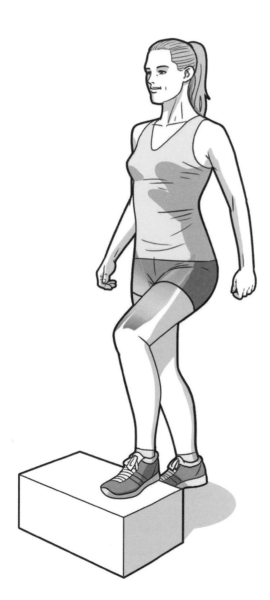

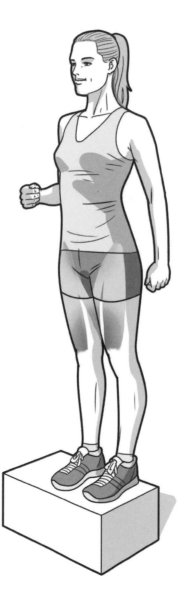

SIDE SKIP SHUFFLE

Side to side movements are a fantastic way to build lateral stability and make your legs more resilient. The side skip shuffle is a great warm up exercise or a good option for including some cardio between strength sets.

INSTRUCTIONS:

Stand sideways at one end of a room or hallway with your feet a little wider than shoulder width apart. Skip to the side by bringing your back foot to your front foot, and then reach out with that front foot. Skip to the side while clicking your heels together between each stride. Skip down to one end of the room, and then return back, still facing the same way so that you're leading with the other leg on your return trip.

PERFORMANCE GOAL:

Aim to complete 15 yards per trip for 20 reps.

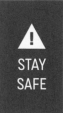

STAY SAFE

While this is a fast-motion exercise, it's not one you want to rush. Moving too quickly increases your risk of tripping or rolling an ankle. When in doubt, slow down the pace and emphasize a smooth, controlled motion.

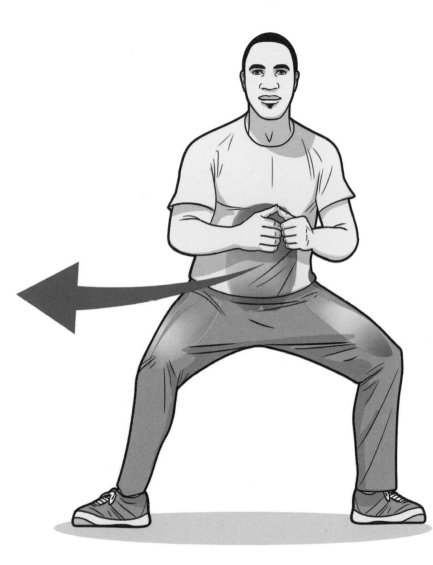

VARIATIONS:

Side skips are usually done with the legs slightly bent, but you can bend your knees and squat with each skip to make the exercise more challenging. You can even turn these into full-on side skip squats if you're really up for a challenge.

GO DEEPER WORKOUT

This workout program integrates the exercises from Level 2. Again, this is a flexible template, so feel free to make any changes or adjustments to fit your level of fitness as well as your preferences.

. . . .

Cardio/Warm-up:

TWO ROUNDS OF:

ISOMETRIC SQUATS 30 seconds (page 66)

STEP-UPS OR SIDE SKIP SHUFFLE 1 minute (pages 70 and 72)

HANGING TUCK 10 to 15 seconds (page 58)

SIDE PLANKS 30 seconds per side (page 64)

Main strength workout:

THREE ROUNDS OF:

SPLIT SQUATS 20 reps per side (page 50)

STANDING CALF RAISES 20 reps (page 62)

WALL-WALKING HANDSTAND Up and down the wall (page 60)

COMPLETE AS MANY REPS AS POSSIBLE WITHIN ONE MINUTE:

FLOOR PUSH-UPS (page 54)

AUSTRALIAN PULL-UPS (page 56)

LYING LEG RAISES (page 48)

LEVEL 3

Power Up

One of the great things about calisthenics is that there's always room to progress. When you're ready to tackle these moves, you'll already have a high level of physical capability. And, even these Level 3 techniques can be developed well beyond the scope of this book.

Remember that you can mix and match these moves with any of the exercises in the previous sections. You're also free to adjust these techniques to fit your body and fitness level. There is a lot of variability in calisthenics and fitness in general, so there's little point in trying to force yourself to do things a certain way. This is especially true if a particular approach compromises your ability to stick to your workout routine because the rules don't align with your body, lifestyle, or fitness level.

Use the exercises in this section as a general guide and as a source of ideas rather than as a strict set of instructions. Creativity and customization will become the norm as you advance in your training career, so have fun with what you're doing and make changes as you grow.

HANGING LEG RAISE

The hanging leg raise is a seemingly simple move that provides multiple benefits. It not only strengthens your abs, hip flexors, arms, and grip, but it is also a good mobility drill for your lower back.

INSTRUCTIONS:

Begin in a tight hang from an overhead support, remembering to keep your arms, back, and core tense. Pull your toes up so that the fronts of your legs are tight as well. Flex your hips to pull your knees up as high as possible while keeping your torso upright. Pause at the top and lower your feet down with control. Keep your feet slightly in front of your body to prevent swinging.

PERFORMANCE GOAL:

Aim to complete three sets of 10 to 15 leg raises, with smooth and controlled reps.

> **⚠ STAY SAFE**
>
> As with the other core exercises, stop if you feel stress in your lower back. Breathe as smoothly as possible to prevent yourself from tiring out and dropping off the bar. Always make sure you're in control during the exercise and land softly on the balls of your feet when finished.

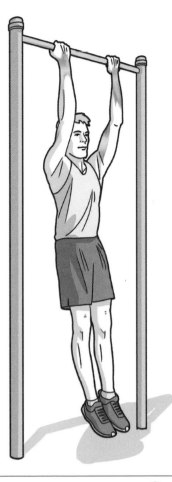

VARIATIONS:

You can adjust the difficulty of this exercise by extending your legs out in front of you. The more you straighten your legs, the more resistance you'll place on your abs and hips.

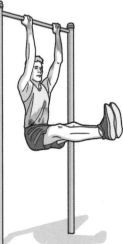

BULGARIAN SPLIT SQUAT

The Bulgarian split squat (or elevated split squat) uses leverage to place more bodyweight onto your front leg. You'll naturally feel your front leg working harder both to push you up as well as to stabilize your hips through a range of motion that is larger than the floor split squat in Level 2 (see page 50).

INSTRUCTIONS:

Set up in the same stance you would use for a standard split squat, except you're now placing your back foot on an elevated surface like a step. Bend your front knee forward to squat down onto your front leg while keeping your hips square and torso upright. Pause at the bottom and push yourself back up with your front leg.

PERFORMANCE GOAL:

Aim to complete three sets of 20 reps on each leg.

> **⚠ STAY SAFE**
>
> Rotating, twisting, and shifting can pull your front leg out of alignment, which not only stresses your joints but also makes the exercise weaker.

VARIATIONS:

This is a great mobility exercise, so work on getting deeper as you become stronger with this technique. You can also add a touch of weight by holding onto something heavy. Just know that a little weight goes a long way, so start off light.

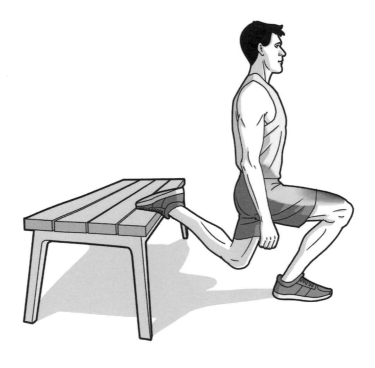

REVERSE PLANK

The reverse plank (or straight-leg hip bridge) targets your hip and posterior chain strength. It quickly exposes any areas you might be neglecting and strengthens them.

INSTRUCTIONS:

Begin by sitting on the floor with your hands slightly behind your hips and your legs straight out in front of you. Pack your shoulders down to push your hands into the floor. At the same time, tense the backs of your legs by pressing into your heels. Use your glutes and hamstrings to drive your hips up until your body forms a straight line. Pause at the top before returning your hips to the floor. Repeat this move or hold the top position for an isometric variation.

PERFORMANCE GOAL:

Aim to complete two sets of 20 reps or hold for one minute.

STAY SAFE Remember to stabilize through your back and lift up using the muscles in the backs of your legs. If you feel your lower back doing all the work, bend your knees to make the exercise easier.

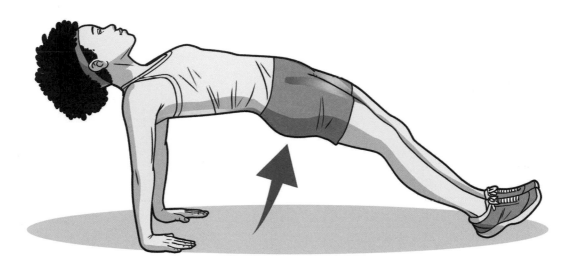

VARIATIONS:

Like the table bridge (see page 52), this technique can be modified by bending or straightening your legs to adjust the length of your body. Bending your knees even slightly will reduce resistance, while locking your knees will maximize it.

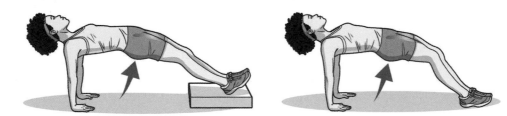

ARCHER PUSH-UP

The archer push-up is the next level of progressive push-up techniques, where you place more of your weight onto a single arm. Eventually, you'll have all of your weight on one arm and be doing one-arm push-ups!

INSTRUCTIONS:

Begin at the top position just as you would when practicing any other push-up (see page 54). Place your main pushing hand under your chest with your assistance arm off to the side, fingers pointing away from you. You may want to place your feet slightly wider than shoulder width. Lower your chest down to touch the back of your pressing hand, then pause at the bottom before pushing yourself back up. Complete the same number of reps on each side.

PERFORMANCE GOAL:

Aim to complete three sets of eight to 12 reps.

STAY SAFE Keep the shoulder of your pressing arm packed down and back at the bottom of each rep to prevent stress in your wrist, elbow, and shoulder joints.

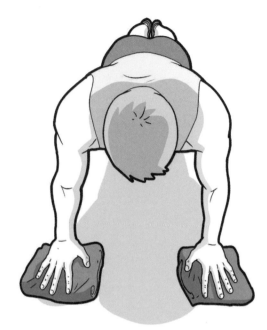

VARIATIONS:

Archer push-ups are easy to adjust; the farther apart your hands are, the more weight you place on the pressing arm. I recommend starting with your hands close together to get a feel for the move before you attempt a more challenging variation.

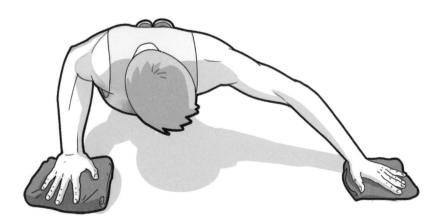

PULL-UP

The full-body pull-up is one of the most intense and complete upper body exercises. It is also one of the safest exercises for your back because it places almost no stress on your spine.

INSTRUCTIONS:

Grab an overhead support with a secure grip and "screw" your arms into your shoulders by turning the point of your elbows forward. Pull your shoulder blades together and drive your elbows down and in toward your sides to lift yourself up. Pause once the top of your chest is at the same height as your hands, and then lower yourself with control.

PERFORMANCE GOAL:

Aim to complete three sets of 15 reps.

⚠️ STAY SAFE	Elbow strain is one of the most common injuries associated with pull-ups. You can prevent this by keeping your shoulder blades together and your arms rotated, so the points of your elbows aim slightly to the front.

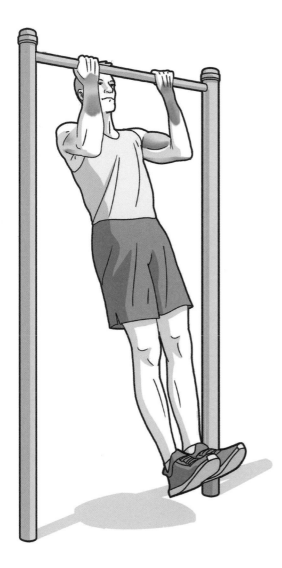

VARIATIONS:

You can make pull-ups easier with a lower body assist like pushing your feet off an elevated surface. You can also make the exercise more difficult by placing your hands closer together, which will challenge your shoulder mobility and grip strength.

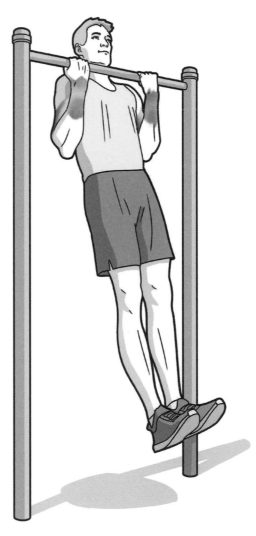

FRONT LEVER

The front lever is often one of the first classic calisthenics moves people become comfortable with. It requires a lot of strength in your arms and back as well as total body stability.

INSTRUCTIONS:

Grab a sturdy support and pick your knees up into a hanging tuck position (see page 58). Lower your hips until they are the same height as your shoulders. From there, extend your legs outward while holding yourself in place with the tension in your back. Hold the position before tucking your legs back in and returning your feet to the floor.

PERFORMANCE GOAL:

Aim to complete two sets, holding the position for 10 seconds per set.

⚠ STAY SAFE	This is one of the safest, yet most intense back exercises in existence. In spite of the safety of this exercise, make sure to continue breathing to prevent dizziness. As always, avoid losing control and letting your feet crash to the floor.

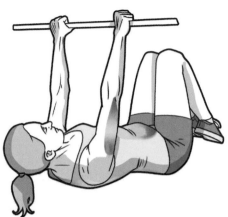

VARIATIONS:

Bend your knees to make this exercise easier. You can also experiment with extending one leg while keeping the other tucked to get a feel for what it's like to stabilize your whole body with your back muscles.

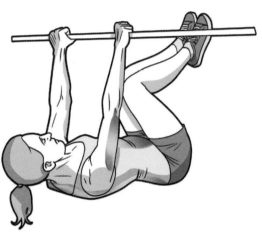

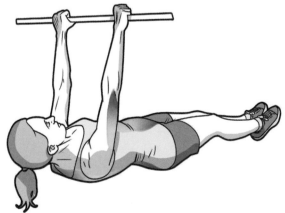

HANDSTAND PUSH-UP

Handstand push-ups require a boatload of shoulder and arm strength, making them an impressive feat.

INSTRUCTIONS:

Walk up the wall to your desired incline to set your resistance. Make sure your hands and feet are even as you keep your core tight. Do not allow your hips to sag. Slowly lower your face down just in front of your hands, pausing about one inch off the floor. Press your whole body up and away from your hands until your arms are straight. Repeat.

PERFORMANCE GOAL:

Aim to complete three sets of three to five reps.

STAY SAFE

Remember to save a little energy in your muscles so you can walk back down the wall with control.

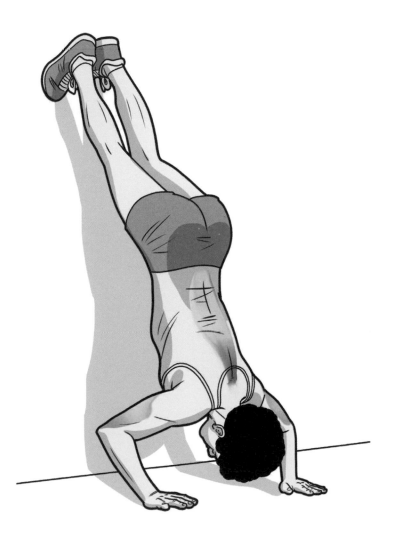

VARIATIONS:

This is a tough move at any angle since you have to either push into the wall or up against gravity, depending on your angle. If you want to make the handstand push-up easier, place your feet on an elevated surface and bend your hips 90 degrees. This will put you in an L shape, and you can do handstand push-ups without working against your full bodyweight.

STARFISH PLANKS

Starfish planks are an advanced lateral chain exercise, building upon the side plank (see page 64) by removing the assistance of your top leg, so the side facing the floor has to work much harder.

INSTRUCTIONS:

Get into a side plank position just like you did in Level 2. Place one foot on top of the other while keeping your body in a straight line from your shoulders to your ankles. Lift your top leg up a few inches while maintaining tension in your back, hips, and supporting leg. Hold before bringing your top leg back down and doing the same thing on the other side.

PERFORMANCE GOAL:

Aim to complete two sets, holding this position for 45 seconds on each side per set.

⚠️ STAY SAFE	Remember to keep your shoulders back and press your weight through your forearm instead of the point of your elbow. This will help prevent strain on your elbow and shoulder joint.

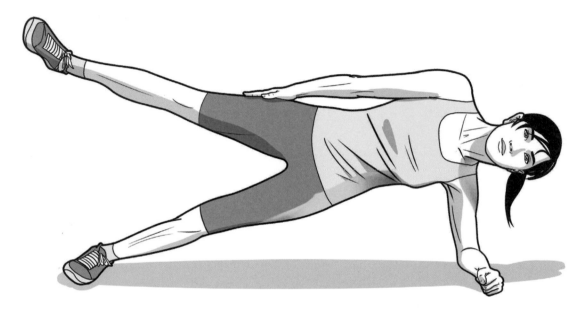

VARIATIONS:

The higher you lift your leg, the more resistance you'll place on the side of your body facing the floor. If you can't quite lift your top leg, you can lift just the heel while keeping the toes of each foot in contact with each other.

SINGLE-LEG CALF RAISES

The single-leg calf raise is one of the strongest calf exercises you can perform, especially when practiced on an elevated surface like a step. Alternate legs with minimal rest between sets for the best results. Just like the calf raises in the Level 2 program (see page 62), remember that while the movement of the exercise happens at the ankle, the rest of the muscles in the leg are active to prevent knee or hip movement.

INSTRUCTIONS:

Stand with both feet on a step with your heels hanging slightly over the edge. Hold on to something sturdy and shift all of your weight onto one leg, making sure to keep your pelvis level and front facing. Lower your supporting heel while maintaining tension throughout your whole leg. Pause and push into the ball of your foot to drive your heel and your whole body straight up. Pause at the top before dropping back down.

PERFORMANCE GOAL:

Aim to complete three sets of 20 reps on each foot.

⚠️ STAY SAFE	Try not to grip the step with your toes. Doing so can cause excessive stress in the bottom of your foot while limiting your range of motion. Keep your toes relaxed and roll on the ball of your foot.

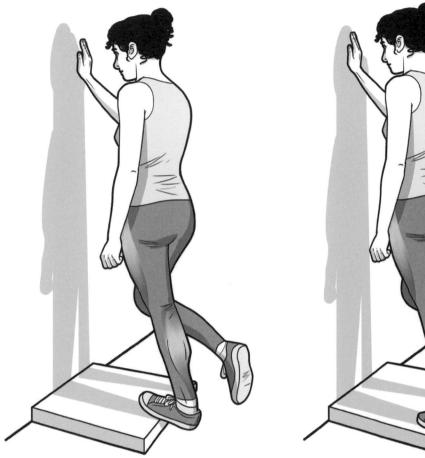
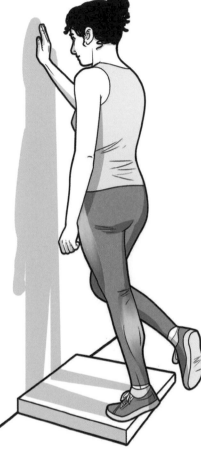

VARIATIONS:

You can make this technique easier or harder, depending on how much assistance you use with your upper body. Leaning onto a support with a tight grip can make this move easier, while only lightly touching a supportive object will make it a significant challenge.

TOWEL HANGS

Towel hangs are just like the tight hang from Level 1 (see page 38), only now you're hanging onto a pair of towels folded over your support. Holding onto the towels adds a new level of challenge to your whole back and arms while also working your grip.

INSTRUCTIONS:

Use a support that you can reach without jumping. Fold two towels over your support, spacing the towels about shoulder width apart. Grab each towel with one hand, ensuring every finger and your thumbs are tightly wrapped around the towels. Gently lift your feet off the floor to apply resistance while keeping your arms, shoulders, and back tight. Hang there before gently bringing your feet back to the floor.

PERFORMANCE GOAL:

Aim to complete two sets, holding the position for 1 minute per set.

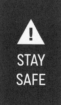

STAY SAFE

Like the tight hang, end your set if you feel any stress or pain in your shoulders or elbows. The same rule now applies to your hands and wrists; this technique will challenge your hands, but it shouldn't hurt them.

VARIATIONS:

Experiment with using towels of various thicknesses. Thicker towels typically provide more of a challenge, while thinner towels provide an easier grip. You can also use multiple towels to increase the thickness of your grip.

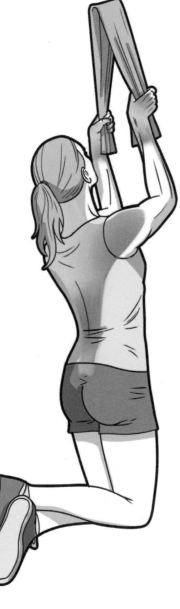

BURPEE

The burpee is the exercise so many of us love to hate because it's one of the best ways to jack your heart rate sky-high.

INSTRUCTIONS:

The traditional burpee is done by squatting down and placing your hands shoulder width in front of you. From there, jump both of your feet back into a plank position and do one push-up (see page 54). At the top of the push-up, hop your feet back to your hands and stand up with enough force to jump into the air with your hands reaching overhead.

The real challenge is in the quality of the reps rather than the number. Like many calisthenics drills, there's a tendency to do burpees for very high reps, which can mean a loss in technical quality. As I've advised with other exercises, your priority should be on the quality of your movements rather than on the quantity or speed of your reps.

PERFORMANCE GOAL:

Aim to complete 15 to 20 reps.

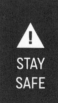

STAY SAFE

Watch out for the tendency to sag your hips to the floor when you push your legs out into the plank position. Maintain a slight arch in your spine to prevent stress on your lower back at the bottom of each rep.

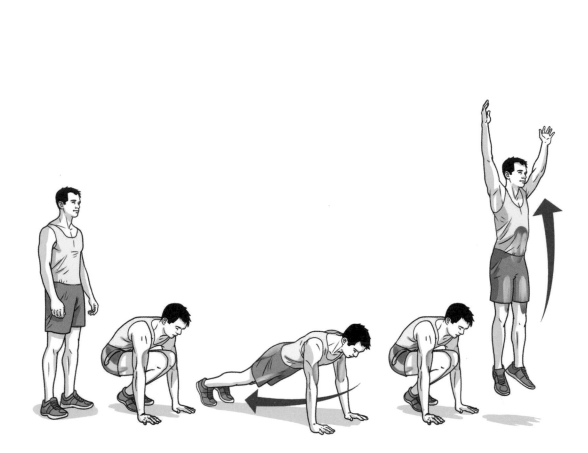

VARIATIONS:

You can omit the push-up if it is a struggle point for you, or you can bring your hands down to an elevated surface, like a weight bench, to make the exercise easier. If you're looking for more challenge, try jumping forward instead of straight up.

SKI HOPS

Ski hops are a simple jumping drill that I like to assign to folks when they are getting ready for ski season. Ski hops build endurance in the lower body in a way that mimics ripping down a bumpy ski run.

INSTRUCTIONS:

Pick a line or seam in the floor and stand just a few inches off to the side of it with your feet close together and your toes pointing slightly toward the line. Hop with both feet about a foot forward, landing on the other side of the line, rotating your feet slightly, so your toes continue to point toward the line. Hop down the line for the length of the room without stopping or pausing.

PERFORMANCE GOAL:

Aim to travel a distance of about 20 to 30 yards or time your sets to be 20 to 30 seconds each.

STAY SAFE

Make sure you keep your knees bent and stay on the balls of your feet. This will allow you to absorb the impact of each landing as well as spring readily into the next jump.

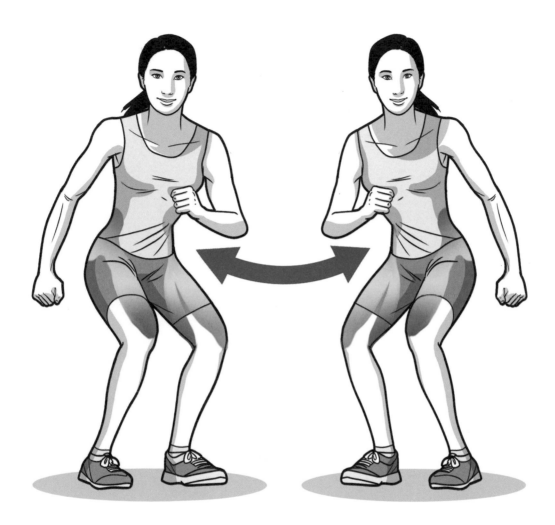

VARIATIONS:

Changing up the width and distance of your jumps is the best way to vary this technique. It's usually best to keep your hops quick and short, but feel free to stretch your jumps out to cover more distance if you are needing more of a challenge.

CROSS-PUNCH WITH FRONT KICKS

This drill builds off the cross-punch exercise from Level 1 (see page 44), only now you're adding a kick with each leg between every set of punches. The kicks will make your legs work harder than they do when you're holding a static stance. This extra challenge will not only elevate your heart rate but also require more stability and coordination.

INSTRUCTIONS:

Begin this drill the same way you start when practicing cross-punches: with your feet wide apart and your knees bent. Do one cross-punch with each arm, and then shift all of your weight onto one leg. Extend the other foot straight out in a front kick. Bend your knee to pull the foot back in and place it on the floor. Then, shift your weight onto that leg and repeat the same process on the other leg. Once you have both legs back on the floor, perform another two punches and repeat. Make sure you return to a wide stance with both knees bent after each kick. This wider stance will make you more stable and reduce stress on your knees while also making the exercise more effective.

PERFORMANCE GOAL:

Aim to complete 25 to 50 reps, where punching with each fist and kicking with each leg counts as one rep.

STAY SAFE — Don't be tempted to rush this exercise since there are a lot of twisting forces at work here. Instead, strive to maintain smooth movements and steady transitions.

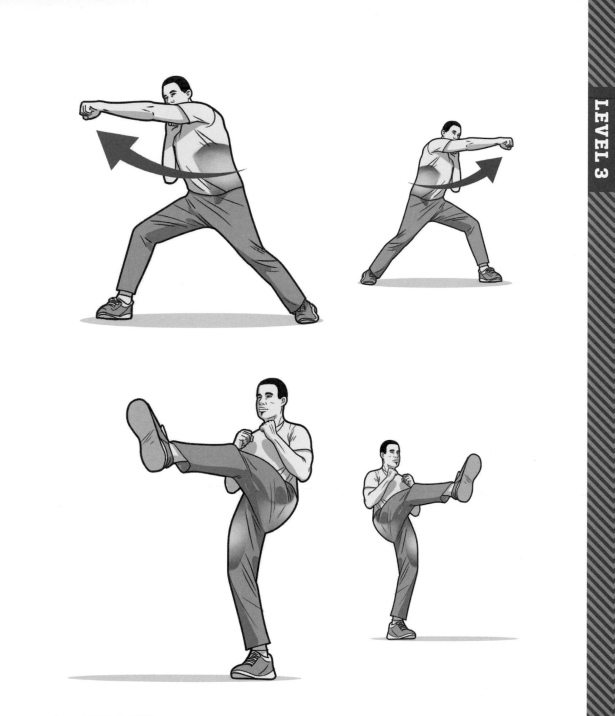

VARIATIONS:

Like with the cross-punch exercise, vary the height of your punches and kicks to bring a unique coordination challenge to your practice.

POWER UP WORKOUT

The basic pattern for this workout uses a combination of heart rate boosting moves along with strength moves to elevate the level of variety and coordination in the workout. As always, feel free to modify this template to suit your fitness needs.

. . . .

Warm-up

TWO ROUNDS OF:

HANGING LEG RAISES 15 reps (page 76)

REVERSE PLANKS 1 minute (page 80)

SKI HOPS 20 to 30 seconds (page 98)

Upper body workout

THREE ROUNDS OF:

ARCHER PUSH-UPS 8 reps per side (page 82)

PULL-UPS 12 reps (page 84)

HANDSTAND PUSH-UPS 5 reps (page 88)

FRONT LEVERS 10 seconds (page 86)

Lower body and core workout

TWO ROUNDS OF:

STARFISH PLANKS 30 seconds per side (page 90)

BULGARIAN SPLIT SQUATS 15 reps per side (page 78)

SINGLE-LEG CALF RAISES 20 reps per side (page 92)

Cardio/Stretch-out

FOUR ROUNDS OF:

BURPEES 15 reps (page 96)

TOWEL HANGS 20 seconds (page 94)

CROSS-PUNCH WITH FRONT KICKS 1 minute (page 100)

CHAPTER THREE

FLEXIBILITY AND RESTORATION

A proper workout is not always about pushing yourself as hard as possible. A workout isn't beneficial only when you stress your body to its limits. In fact, some of the most effective training methods you can practice will actually help reduce stress on your body and mind.

Recovery exercises, like the ones in this chapter, offer you the chance to let your mind and body "downshift" from a sympathetic state to a parasympathetic state. This helps your body—primarily your nervous system—return to a more neutral state where your heart rate is normal and your mind is calm.

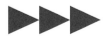

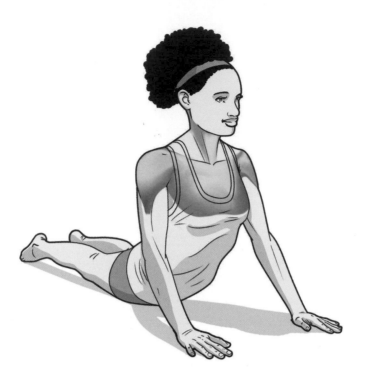

Cool Down Stretches

Taking time to cool down is like landing an airplane after a long flight. Failing to practice recovery methods is akin to taking your plane up in the sky, and then just letting it drop whenever it runs out of gas. While it is possible to skip your cool down exercises, practicing them ensures that you remain in control, so you're less likely to crash later on.

These techniques are especially important in our hectic modern lives where we seldom take the time to relax and rejuvenate. Practicing these simple strategies can do wonders to ease your physical and mental stress, which not only helps you recover from your hard workouts but from hard days at work as well.

The following recommendations apply to each of the suggested cool down stretches:

PERFORMANCE GOAL:

Aim to complete one to two sets, holding each stretch for 20 to 30 seconds per set.

> ⚠️ **STAY SAFE**
>
> Stretching is meant to be a therapeutic form of exercise and not something you should force. Ease into each stretch until you feel a light pull on the targeted muscles. Hold the light stretch while breathing smoothly.

VARIATIONS:

Experiment with slight variations in your hand and foot placements. Adjusting the height or width of your hands and feet can improve your stability and help you emphasize the targeted muscles.

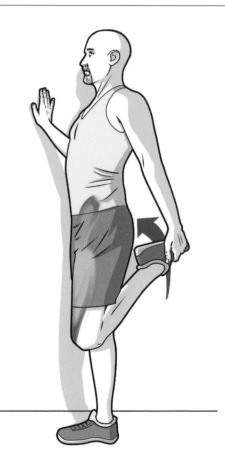

STANDING QUAD STRETCH

The standing quad stretch is one of the best ways to stretch out the muscles in the front of your thighs and hips. It's a particularly useful way to release stiffness that accumulates after sitting for long periods of time.

INSTRUCTIONS:

For stability and safety, practice this stretch while holding onto something sturdy like a tree or post. Shift all of your weight onto the leg that's closest to your supporting hand.

Bring your other foot up behind your hip by bending your knee as much as possible, pulling your foot close to your pelvis with the hand that is not holding on to your support. From there, gently push the knee of your bent leg backward until you feel a light stretch in the front of your leg. After holding, bring your knee forward to release the stretch. Let go of your foot and turn your body to face the other direction to repeat on the other side.

Be sure to maintain an upright posture without bending forward or leaning back. It's important to keep your hips square; don't twist or tilt your pelvis during the stretch. If you have trouble bringing your foot up to your hips, you can place it on an elevated surface behind you like a bench or chair.

HANDS CLASP BEHIND STRETCH

This is one of my favorite moves to relieve stress in your upper body and stretch out the front of your shoulders. It also promotes good posture and "opens your chest" to improve breathing.

INSTRUCTIONS:

Begin by standing with a tall posture, feet shoulder width apart. Reach behind your back and clasp the fingers of both hands together. Take a deep breath in and use your back muscles to pull your shoulders down and back as you push your hands together. Hold the stretch before gently letting go of your hands to release. Roll your shoulders a few times to shake out any tension in your upper body.

You can make this stretch easier or harder depending on how you hold onto your hands behind your back. Beginners may find they have to grasp their fingertips or keep their hands pretty open at first. Over time, you should be able to fully clasp your hands together with your palms touching. For the most advanced version, press your palms together without holding on to your hands at all, using only your back muscles to produce the stretch.

SEATED TOE PULLS

The seated toe pull stretches almost every muscle along your backside. It's also a lot more effective than just bending over and trying to touch your toes since you, rather than gravity, are in control of the tension.

INSTRUCTIONS:

Begin by sitting on the floor with your legs straight out in front of you. Bend your knees and reach your hands forward, so you can get a firm grip on the balls of your feet. You may find it easier to get a grip if you're wearing shoes.

Gently straighten your legs until you feel a light stretch in your hamstrings. Once you're there, press the balls of your feet forward to further stretch your back. Make sure to breathe normally as you hold this stretch. Pull your toes back to release the stretch and gently shake out any tension along your hamstrings.

This is a very easy stretch to control since the farther you push out your feet, the greater your stretch will be. You can also try reaching diagonally across with either your right hand to your left foot or vice versa to get a twisting back and lat stretch.

SEATED TWIST

The seated twist can do wonders for releasing tension that may be hiding along your spine, hips, and shoulders. It's also a great way to stretch tight muscles in your neck, which can be a source of tension headaches.

INSTRUCTIONS:

Begin sitting on the floor with both legs straight out in front of you. Bend one knee and place that foot on the outside of the other leg (which remains flat on the floor). Twist your torso toward your bent knee and place the opposite arm on the outside of the knee. You may want to place the other hand behind you for stability and to assist with holding your torso upright rather than letting it hunch over. Turn your head to look in the direction you're twisting while continuing to breathe. Stop pressing your arm against your knee to release the stretch gently. Repeat on the other side.

There are several ways to adjust this technique, including modifying how much you bend your knee or how far you twist. As with any stretch, don't force it to the point of pain. Rather, hold a light stretch while taking deep breaths.

SIT-BACKS

This stretch is a fantastic technique to loosen up your lats while also decompressing your spine. It simulates a hanging motion without requiring as much strength from the upper body and with easier means for adjusting the intensity.

INSTRUCTIONS:

Begin the stretch standing upright and holding onto a set of suspension straps or a sturdy railing. Bend your knees and sit back with your hips, so you form a straight line between your hands and your hips. Keep your weight flat on your feet and breathe deeply as you let your shoulders lift up by your ears. Push your hips forward to stand up out of the stretch and roll your shoulders to shake out any tension.

If you are using a suspension trainer, you can emphasize one side of your back by gently twisting your torso. If you're using a stable bar, shift your weight side to side to help stretch out one side, and then the other. The more you shift your weight, the deeper the stretch will be. Experiment with both the isometric and dynamic versions of this stretch. Twist and hold for a deep isometric stretch, or twist side to side in a smooth motion to increase blood flow and work the stiffness out of your muscles.

STANDING ARM PULL

The standing arm pull is a great compliment to the sit-back stretch (see page 112), as it addresses the front of the shoulder and arm.

INSTRUCTIONS:

Begin the stretch by finding a sturdy upright support like a post or the edge of a wall. Stand slightly in front of the support and reach behind you to place the palm of your closest hand on the support slightly below shoulder level. Use a reverse stance, placing the opposite foot of the arm that's on the post in front of you with your feet shoulder width apart. Gently twist your torso away from the post to create a stretch in your arm, shoulder, and chest. Hold before gently twisting back to release the stretch. Switch feet and face the other way to repeat on the other side.

The standing arm pull—like many other stretches—requires you to apply a bit of strength to facilitate the stretch. This promotes tension control and stability, but you have to be careful not to force the stretch as far as possible. Apply just enough tension to create a moderate stretch without feeling like you're trying to pull your arm out of its shoulder socket.

STANDING OVERHEAD SIDE REACH

This stretch is a great example of the fact that, sometimes, simple is best. In its simplicity, this stretch is ideal as a workday move to ease stress and tension after hours of sitting at a desk.

INSTRUCTIONS:

The setup is very basic; stand with your feet shoulder width apart and your shoulders back. Reach up with one arm as high as you can without straining your arm or shoulder. Allow your hips to shift a few inches so that you are leaning gently to the side with your lowered fingers reaching toward the floor. At the same time, gently reach your raised hand overhead, stretching in the direction you are bending. This should create a stretch along the whole side of your body, especially along your back and obliques. Breathe smoothly. Shift your hips back to neutral to release the stretch. Repeat on the other side.

You can practice this stretch in both isometric and dynamic fashions, just remember to move in a smooth motion, so you don't pull or strain your muscles. This is meant to be a gentle stretch rather than an aerobic workout.

It's also tempting to twist yourself to the side as you reach overhead. It's not harmful to twist, but it can compromise the stretch you're trying to achieve.

LYING FRONT STRETCH

This unique stretch works the backside of your body while stretching the front. It's also an effective way to practice extending your upper spine, a skill sorely lacking in our sit-and-slouch society.

INSTRUCTIONS:

Begin by lying front-side down on the floor with your arms bent to place your hands near your chest. Lift your chin up off the floor, looking forward while tucking your shoulder blades down and back away from your ears. Gently press your palms into the floor to lift your chest and extend your back. Press yourself up until you either feel a light stretch along your front side or until you've reached the limit for how far you can lift. Hold while breathing as deeply as possible, then gently lower your torso back to the floor.

While performing this stretch, tense the muscles along your posterior chain, including your hamstrings, glutes, and spinal erectors. Doing so will help the stress flow along your whole body rather than pooling in a sensitive spot. The most common pinch point for this stretch is the lower back. If you feel stress building in your back, lower your torso a few inches or until you no longer feel any strain.

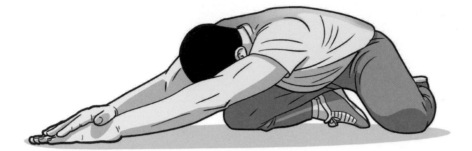

Restorative Poses

These poses are meant to help your muscles and nervous system wind down after your intense workouts. This wind down time is a vital yet often over-looked part of an effective workout. Our busy lives make it all too tempting to finish a workout, and then rush to complete the next item on our to-do list. I don't recommend ending your workout in such a sudden manner. When you finish your workout without winding down, your nervous system remains in sympathetic dominance, which promotes your body's fight-or-flight instincts—a stressful state in which to spend the rest of your day.

Practicing these poses for just a few minutes at the end of your workout helps downshift your system into a parasympathetic state. These poses reduce stress and promote faster recovery. They may not look like much, but they can have a large influence in your overall health and well-being.

CHILD'S POSE

The child's pose is a staple in restorative yoga for good reason. It places your upper body in an elongated position, which helps with breathing, while passively stretching your lower back and hips.

INSTRUCTIONS:

Set up for this pose on your hands and knees. Place your feet and knees close together and spread your hands shoulder width apart. Point your toes back, so your feet are resting on the instep. If this is uncomfortable, you can practice this stretch on a towel or mat to reduce pressure points.

Sit your hips back onto your feet while keeping your hands in place, so your arms stretch out in front of you. Exhale as you do this to allow your spine to round slightly. Hold the position and continue to breathe as deeply as possible. When you're finished, gently pull your hands toward your torso and push yourself up into a seated kneeling position.

VARIATIONS:

If you have trouble sitting back onto your heels, you may want to spread your knees apart so you can sink down between your legs. You can also offer additional assistance by placing a support, like a yoga block, under your hips.

LYING FRONT POSE WITH FULL BELLY BREATHING

Deep belly breathing is an effective way to switch from a sympathetic dominant nervous system to a parasympathetic dominant system. Unfortunately, such deep breathing is becoming more uncommon as our busy lifestyles leave us prone to shallow chest breathing. Practicing this deep breathing technique after each workout can do wonders for your overall stress levels.

INSTRUCTIONS:

Lie front-side down, placing your arms where they are most comfortable: by your sides, stretched overhead, or extended out to the side. Find a completely relaxed position so that you feel like you're melting into the floor. You can turn your head to either side, but I find it's best to place something soft under your forehead, so you can maintain a neutral neck.

Once you're in position, begin the breathing exercise by inhaling as deep a breath as possible through your nose. As you breathe in, allow your torso to expand in every direction, including out to the sides, into the floor, and even up and down to slightly elongate your spine. Let your breath release as you exhale in a relaxed manner instead of forcefully blowing out. Continue for as many breaths as you'd like.

LYING CHAIR POSE

The lying chair pose is just like the lying front pose (see page 118), only now you're facing up with your back against the floor and your knees bent to bring some elevation to your legs.

INSTRUCTIONS:

You can practice this by either bending your knees with your feet flat on the floor or by placing your legs up on a chair. Elevating your legs improves relaxation in the lower body and decompresses your hips, knees, and ankles. It's a particularly relaxing posture after a hard leg workout or long hike.

Make sure to focus on drawing your breath as deep into your belly as possible to release any tension you may be holding in your core muscles. Hold the breath for one second before exhaling in a relaxed manner. I find it helps to imagine a deflating balloon as your body relaxes and releases any tension in your hands, feet, and face during the exhalation. Continue breathing as long as you wish. When you're done, roll over to one side and gently get off the floor. Be careful not to stand up too quickly, which can make you feel dizzy.

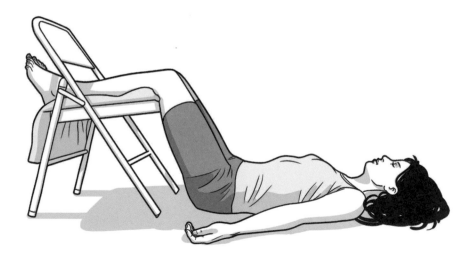

HEALTHY HABITS AND MINDSET

The exercises in this chapter are a great reminder that fitness is not always about stressing you out. Many of the healthiest habits you can practice involve *removing* stress from your mind and body rather than the other way around.

Yes, training can be a real challenge, and sure, there are going to be times where you'll be pushing yourself outside of your comfort zone. However, such occasions are supposed to be the exception rather than the norm. Acute, short-term moments of stress can stimulate change. On the other hand, chronic mental and physical stress will depress that stimulus and prevent your body from changing very much at all.

To avoid overstressing yourself, and to keep your training fresh for both mind and body, I recommend changing up how you practice your exercises. You don't have to use a different routine every workout; but play around with some of the variations I mentioned for each technique.

It's also crucially important to avoid treating exercise as a form of punishment. You cannot abuse yourself into shape with workouts that always leave you feeling exhausted and depleted. Some experts recommend "leaving a little in the tank" after each workout, and I fully endorse this idea.

This goes for mental training as well. No one ever accomplished more in life by constantly berating themselves with negative self-talk. If anything, the opposite is the case. I'll discuss this notion more in the following chapter.

CHAPTER FOUR

ONWARD

A truly effective approach to exercise requires more than hard work and effort in the gym. There's another aspect of self-care and recovery that's just as important as the actual exercises you practice.

In this chapter, I'll be covering some of the essential points that will balance out your physical training, including tips for healthy approaches toward self-care as well as guidance for building your own workout plan with a sample of a productive workout log.

Remember that the aspects of self-care discussed in this chapter are some of the most commonly neglected aspects of a successful work-out plan. Paying attention to these topics can accelerate your results while also making your training a lot more enjoyable.

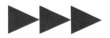

REST AND SELF-AWARENESS

In fitness, stress is like medicine. In the right doses, stress stimulates health and progress. However, if you get the dose wrong, stress can poison both body and mind and break your results rather than make them. That's why the following tips are so important; they will help you ensure that the stress you experience from your training will stimulate the changes you want rather than prevent them from happening.

The first important aspect of health and recovery is rest. Your body doesn't change during your workouts; it changes—grows stronger, more flexible, and more fit—in recovery. Therefore, if you hardly rest, you'll severely compromise your results.

Sleep is the biggest component of rest. It's so important that I often tell people that improving their sleep habits can be more beneficial to their fitness goals than improving their diet and exercise program combined. Getting proper sleep should always be as high a priority as sticking to your diet and exercise habits. If you're struggling to make progress and running on little rest, I promise getting enough sleep will help.

Aside from sleep, resting from a particular activity is also important. Going all-out in your workouts every day inhibits recovery; allowing your muscles to rest a bit after your workouts is essential for building strength and muscle. A balanced, varied program will let your various muscle groups rest after high-fatigue workouts.

Recovery also includes mental and emotional rest. Meditation, relaxing, and just plain having fun are not luxuries. They are essential elements in your health and should be pursued on a daily basis. Make time to blow off steam and do something that feels good. Sing and dance to your favorite song as you drive home from work. Take a walk along the local nature trail or in the park during your lunch break. Talk to a friend about something other than work.

When we speak of rest and recovery as part of a balanced, healthy lifestyle, pain management is another important aspect to consider. The two primary types of pain are superficial and internal pain. Superficial pain is skin deep, like cuts, burns, and blisters. In calisthenics, the most common superficial injuries are to the hands and feet. Often, you can avoid or address these injuries with properly fitting apparel or gloves. You may find that applying a regular moisturizer can help prevent cracked skin if you live in a dry climate. Skin softener helps a lot with the callouses that tend to build up through calisthenics practice, especially with pulling techniques. It's best to avoid any surfaces or grips that aggravate an existing injury to allow your hands time to heal. As you build a regular calisthenics practice, your skin will toughen up over time, helping prevent further superficial injuries.

Internal pain is a much more serious issue, often showing up in the joints, ligaments, and tendons. You can usually identify tendon pain in the form of a sharp and burning sensation around a joint, especially when the joint is under a load. Tendon pain often occurs in joints that have little muscular support like the knees, elbows, and wrists. Pain in these areas should always be addressed and never "worked through" or ignored. Doing so only leads to a greater degree of internal damage, often requiring more serious measures to address it in the future.

Sometimes, a random ache in a joint is merely a tweak where something zigged instead of zagged during your workout. In these cases, the issue should go away after a week or two of rest and light movement to promote blood flow to the area. Applying heat can also improve blood flow and aid in healing.

If pain lasts more than a couple weeks, that's usually a sign that there's a misalignment or imbalance causing stress to build up where it shouldn't. In that case, it's best to get the problem checked out by a professional—an athletic trainer, doctor, or physical therapist—who can assess and help treat the injury. Very often, the exercise you are doing when you feel the pain isn't causing the problem but rather exposing it. So, avoiding that painful technique can offer temporary relief but might not address the underlying issue, which has the potential to continue to worsen over time.

The most important thing to remember is that your healthy habits should improve how you feel. They should make you feel happier, more motivated, more energized, and should reduce pain. If you start to experience chronic fatigue, pain, or a general loss of motivation, there's a good chance something is having a detrimental influence on your mind and body and should be addressed as soon as possible.

DEALING WITH SELF-DOUBT AND FRUSTRATION

The biggest threats to your training success are not physical but rather mental and emotional. Sometimes, mental obstacles can be more detrimental to your goals than even a serious injury.

Few things will hold you back like self-doubt. A lack of faith in your ability to succeed can drain you of motivation while tempting you to look for reasons to quit. Self-doubt is a normal part of any growth process. Anytime you're trying to improve your life, you're venturing into uncharted waters, and there's no telling what you may encounter along your journey. It's perfectly normal to feel like you're not quite sure about what you're doing or what might happen. That's actually a very good sign that you're pushing yourself and expanding your horizons.

On the other side of self-doubt is frustration. While self-doubt prevents you from taking action, frustration comes after you take action and are disappointed with the results. The best thing to do is use your frustration as a springboard to propel you forward. Take stock of just how far you've come and recognize that even making a little progress is 100 percent better than no progress at all. You can also identify areas you may not be addressing, like sleep, diet, or technique, and see if there are some simple things you can do move forward.

Motivation is just like your physical energy level. It's natural for it to ebb and flow with highs and lows throughout life. Sometimes, you may have low motivation for a few days. Other times, you may have low motivation for weeks or even months at a time.

The good news is that while motivation can—and will—leave you, it will also come back. This is why it's important to continue with your training habits, even during times when motivation starts to wane. If you quit or take a long break, you'll lose a lot of ground and be forced to make it all up when the next motivation wave comes in.

It's okay to scale back in your habits when you no longer have the time or motivation to push as hard as you can. Cut back on your training volume or loosen your diet up a bit. You don't have to stay perfect or even do everything "right" all the time to continue making progress. You only need to continue doing what you can, so you're able to ramp back up later.

BUILDING YOUR OWN WORKOUTS

Creating your own workout program can seem like a daunting task, especially when you're starting out. Fear not, my friend. One of the best things about starting out is that this is the easiest time in your training career to make progress. Keep the following points in mind, and you'll be good to go.

The first thing to do is to clearly establish your goals so that you can build your training plan accordingly. Refer back to the material in the first chapter if you need a reminder about how to set your goals and what eating and exercise habits will move you in the right direction. Remember that if you want to burn fat, you'll make burning calories your primary objective. If building muscle is your goal, you'll want to challenge the strength and work capacity of your muscles. And if functional ability is your goal, you'll want to make sure your training is challenging the specific functional capabilities you want to improve.

The next step is to plan out a typical training week. Write your workout schedule onto a weeklong calendar. For the sake of simplicity, I recommend starting with three full-body calisthenics workouts per week. Plan these workouts for nonconsecutive days like Monday, Wednesday, and Friday. This basic template is effective for nearly any objective and has a long history of helping a variety of people find success, from professional athletes to weekend warriors and senior citizens.

The final step, once you have built a weeklong schedule that will work for you, is to decide what exercises you will include in each workout you'll be practicing that week. In the case of your calisthenics training, consider starting with the workout recipes I've given you for each of the three workout levels. Practice the Start Strong routine (see page 46) for at least a few weeks, and move up as you feel ready.

The most important thing at the start is to get in the habit of working and to establish consistency. Aside from that, focus on making sure that your workouts are pointing you toward your goals. If burning fat is your goal, your schedule should include some sort of physical activity most days of the week to maximize calories burned. You'll certainly burn fat with calisthenics training, but you'll also want to supplement with other activities of your choice to keep moving and burning.

If the goal that you established is to build muscle, a three day a week plan will cover your bases, and you'll want to rest on the other days to recover. In this case, plan each of your workouts to challenge your muscles pretty hard, usually with two to four sets of five to 20 reps.

Lastly, if you're working to improve a functional ability, your three day a week strength training plan will supplement your daily skill practice, be it hitting a golf ball or throwing a side kick.

Overall, don't stress about your routine. Your routine should establish enough structure that you can be intentional and thoughtful about approaching your goals but not so rigid that it doesn't actually work with your life. The true key ingredient for your success isn't the nitty-gritty of the routine—it is being consistent with your exercise plan so that you improve from one workout to the next.

WORKOUT LOG

Your workout success doesn't come from the exercises you do or the routine you practice. It comes from *progressing* the exercises you do and the routine you practice. One of the most reliable ways to ensure you're making progress is to keep a workout log.

Keeping a log is pretty simple; just jot down what you've done and any details pertaining to how you did it. I recommend finding a format that is convenient for you. Some people prefer keeping their journal in a simple lined notebook, while others prefer to use a computerized spreadsheet. Personally, I use a simple notepad app on my smartphone, so I always have it with me.

Here's an example of a workout log and the kind of information you should include.

	ACTIVITY	SETS/REPS	GOALS
MON	Ran to the park	1.5 miles, 8 min pace	Jog in place at stoplights
	Incline push-ups on park bench	12 reps / 12 / 10	Try for 12 reps for all 3 sets
	Split squats	15/side / 15/side	Add one more set; try to keep front heel down more
	Ran home	1.5 mile, 8 min pace	Stretch hamstrings afterward
TUE			
WED			
THU			
FRI			
SAT			
SUN			

The second step is the most important. After making a note of what you've done, consider what you can do in your next workout to progress your training. This can be anything from adding a few reps to improving your technique. Jotting down these notes and reflections provides you with a set of directions for what to do in your next workout to continue advancing toward your goals.

There are a few blank logs in the back of this book (see page 131) to help you get started. Use these blank workout logs to develop the habit of keeping a workout journal and to experiment with what format is most convenient for you.

TAKE CARE AND HAVE FUN

Congratulations, my friend, on reaching the end of this book! This may be the last page, but your calisthenics career is just getting started. A plethora of opportunities and possibilities are out there for you to discover, and I'm always here to help you along your journey.

As you continue your training, please keep a few things in mind. First, exercise and physical training are meant to make you feel good and improve your quality of life. If you ever find that your quality of health and life are eroding, please stop and reconsider your approach. Fitness habits that compromise your well-being are neither healthy nor productive.

Second, listen to your body and trust your instincts. Diet and exercise are far from an exact science; even the leading experts don't have all of the answers. If you feel that making a change in your approach may be a good idea, then it is worth acting on that instinct.

Lastly, know that you'll learn far more from personal experience than from any book. Resources like this and the others listed in the back of the book (see page 141), are great places to get ideas, but the real source of knowledge and understanding is to take massive action. Make your plan and take your first step. Where you go from there is up to you, and I'm sure it's going to be a fun and rewarding lifelong journey.

Be fit and live free!

BLANK WORKOUT LOGS

	ACTIVITY	REPS/SETS	GOALS
example:	Incline pushups	3 sets : 12 reps / 12 / 10	Try 12 reps on all 3 sets
MON			
TUE			
WED			
THU			
FRI			
SAT			
SUN			

	ACTIVITY	REPS/SETS	GOALS
example:	Incline pushups	3 sets : 12 reps / 12 / 10	Try 12 reps on all 3 sets
MON			
TUE			
WED			
THU			
FRI			
SAT			
SUN			

	ACTIVITY	REPS/SETS	GOALS
example:	Incline pushups	3 sets : 12 reps / 12 / 10	Try 12 reps on all 3 sets
MON			
TUE			
WED			
THU			
FRI			
SAT			
SUN			

	ACTIVITY	REPS/SETS	GOALS
example:	Incline pushups	3 sets : 12 reps / 12 / 10	Try 12 reps on all 3 sets
MON			
TUE			
WED			
THU			
FRI			
SAT			
SUN			

	ACTIVITY	REPS/SETS	GOALS
example:	Incline pushups	3 sets : 12 reps / 12 / 10	Try 12 reps on all 3 sets
MON			
TUE			
WED			
THU			
FRI			
SAT			
SUN			

	ACTIVITY	REPS/SETS	GOALS
example:	Incline pushups	3 sets : 12 reps / 12 / 10	Try 12 reps on all 3 sets
MON			
TUE			
WED			
THU			
FRI			
SAT			
SUN			

	ACTIVITY	REPS/SETS	GOALS
example:	Incline pushups	3 sets : 12 reps / 12 / 10	Try 12 reps on all 3 sets
MON			
TUE			
WED			
THU			
FRI			
SAT			
SUN			

	ACTIVITY	REPS/SETS	GOALS
example:	Incline pushups	3 sets : 12 reps / 12 / 10	Try 12 reps on all 3 sets
MON			
TUE			
WED			
THU			
FRI			
SAT			
SUN			

RESOURCES

www.reddeltaproject.com is my personal website, where you'll also find my podcast and YouTube videos on calisthenics training and practical fitness solutions.

www.schoolofcalisthenics.com is an expansive Internet resource for learning both basic and advanced calisthenics skills to take your training to the next level.

www.dragondoor.com is the home of the kettlebell and progressive calisthenics revolution; you'll find loads of books, articles, and other resources to make your training fun and supremely effective.

www.monkii.co makes some of the highest quality portable calisthenics training equipment in the world. It's innovative, versatile, and built to last a lifetime.

www.calimove.com hosts some of the most practical calisthenics training programs and videos on the internet.

www.jgcalisthenics.co.uk/home is the online resource of Jake Gay, who's been documenting the beginning of his calisthenics career and his impressive results.

www.spri.com is one of the most popular sources for training equipment for both home and commercial gym use.

www.ringtraining.com is the ultimate resource for innovative gymnastics ring equipment that will add challenge and variety to your calisthenics training.

www.precisionnutrition.com/blog is one of the leading sources for effective, down-to-earth information on nutrition without the dogmatic hype and fads.

www.strongerbyscience.com is a great resource if you want to dive deeper into the latest research on strength training and nutrition.

EXERCISE LIBRARY

INDEX

ACKNOWLEDGMENTS

This book would simply not have been possible without the patient instruction and mentorship of the crew over at DragonDoor.com including Paul Wade, Al and Danny Kavadlo, Adrienne Harvey, and my tae kwon do instructor Grand Master Stephen Barret.

   I also want to thank all of my fellow coaches and trainers, who've taught me more than I could ever learn on my own.

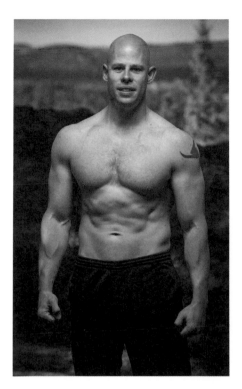

ABOUT THE AUTHOR

Matt Schifferle is a certified calisthenics coach in Denver, Colorado, as well as a team leader for the Dragon Door Progressive Calisthenics Certification. He is the founder of the Red Delta Project: a collection of YouTube videos, podcasts, and books about bodyweight training and diet-free healthy eating. His approach to fitness has helped thousands of people discover how to use healthy habits to enhance their quality of life rather than compromise it.

In his free time, Matt enjoys mountain biking and skiing in the backcountry and finishing the adventure off with a good IPA from a local brewery.